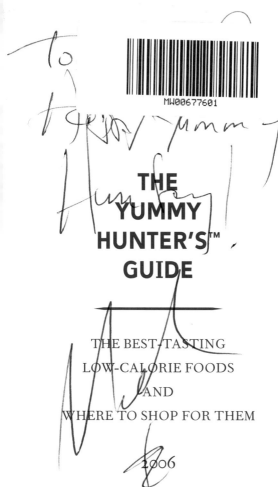

THE YUMMY HUNTER'S™ GUIDE

THE BEST-TASTING

LOW-CALORIE FOODS

AND

WHERE TO SHOP FOR THEM

2006

HELEN BRAND AND
ERIC ROBESPIERRE

ROMAX
PUBLISHING
www.romaxpublishing.com

For information, address
Romax Publishing
P.O. Box 2290
Halesite, NY 11743

Visit our website at www.romaxpublishing.com

PRINTED IN THE UNITED STATES

Library of Congress Cataloging-in-Publication Data

2006 EDITION
Library of Congress Control Number: 2005905665

ISBN-13: 978-0-9755096-1-6
ISBN-10: 0-9755096-1-6

CONTENTS

PREFACE
TO THE 2006 EDITION

Iᴛ ɪs ᴡɪᴛʜ ᴀ sᴇɴsᴇ ᴏꜰ sᴀᴛɪsꜰᴀᴄᴛɪᴏɴ that we are publishing the second edition of *The Yummy Hunter's Guide*. Although we had confidence in the quality of our work and its potential popularity, we could not have expected what an impact our book would make on the lives of those who have used it in conjunction with their diet plans.

As exciting as the first book was, we think the 2006 edition is even better. Jammed packed with 670+ delcious products, of which 254 are new, the 2006 edition provides an even greater selection of foods that will make your diet regimes that much more successful.

We've taken a few products out, either because they're no longer being produced or because they've been replaced by better-tasting, low-cal versions.

The plentiful array of new and delicious low-cal products is a sign that food manufacturers are listening to your demands and are rushing to satisfy your desires.

Over the past year we have seen our Yummy Hunters move away from low-carb products and show a much greater interest in products that are low in fat, that is heart smart. To accommodate this trend, we have marked all low-fat foods, those with 5 grams of fat or less per serving, with an asterisk.

The 2005 Yummy Hunter's Guide has attracted a great deal of media attention. TV, radio, magazine and newspaper exposure has created even more awareness and brought our message to larger audiences, helping greater numbers of dieters to lead healthier and more productive lives.

We would like to say thank you to all the Yummy Hunters out there who purchased our book, sent in new product recommendations, and e-mailed us their success stories.

When the guide was in its final stages, we chose several dieters to use the book. One dieter's story that really hit home was Lauren's. You can read her story on the following pages. It's stories like hers that excite and empower us.

HELEN BRAND
ERIC ROBESPIERRE

P.S. Though we appreciate all your invitations and though, we love to go out and meet all our Yummy Hunters, please do not invite us to another all-you-can-eat, deep-dish apple pie fest.

LAUREN'S STORY

Two years ago, I went to an amusement park with my two children. During this period, I weighed close to 270 pounds.

In public I always felt people were staring at me and laughing about how fat I was. I had a difficult time looking people in the eye. Emotionally, I was dying inside. I felt like a failure. I talked myself into believing I couldn't accomplish anything if I didn't have the strength and determination to stop the weight from piling on.

When my kids wanted to ride on the roller coaster, I had to cram my body in sideways and could barely buckle the belt. The ride attendant told me that maybe I wouldn't be able to take the ride, seeing as I wasn't properly seated. I looked at all the people standing around staring at me and I felt like the fattest person in the world. It was the most humiliating experience of my life. I began to cry. When the attendant saw the tears in my eyes, he went ahead and started the ride.

That two-minute ride was the longest and most uncomfortable ride I have ever been on in my life. I was so twisted in my seat that every bump was excruciatingly painful. In the middle of the ride I promised myself that I would lose weight.

I heard about *The Yummy Hunter's Guide* from a friend. When I learned they were looking for a dieter to try the products in the book before it went to print, I felt this was an opportunity that I couldn't pass up.

As it turned out, *The Yummy Hunter's Guide* was a lifesaver. For the first time in my life I was able to successfully stay on my diet and reach my goals.

Instead of being overwhelmed by the task of finding low-calorie foods that taste good, I now had a powerful shopping resource to help guide me through my diet journey.

Using the foods in *The Yummy Hunter's Guide*, I was able to plan breakfast, lunch and dinner menus. With so many choices, I had plenty of variation and enough great-tasting foods to keep me motivated and to help me lose weight.

I was able to lose 110 pounds! Now I feel good inside, which is the most important thing. I know I have the strength and determination to accomplish anything I want because losing weight has got to be one of the most difficult things to do in the world.

I move differently now. I smile more and look people in the eye. I love to tell people how much weight I have lost. They are always interested in knowing how I did it, and I always tell them about *The Yummy Hunter's Guide* because it's all about eating the right foods.

FOREWORD

Pssst . . . Can i take you for a walk down memory lane? Over the years there was the popcorn diet, the grapefruit diet, the cabbage soup diet and a zillion other diets. Everyone knows the seafood diet. We "see food" and we eat it. Let's face it. We just loooove to eat! Who could blame us, with an abundant amount of options to choose from?

Despite the plethora of diets available today, there is a scarcity of scientific research on their health effects. Most of us run around from dawn to dusk with minimal time to cook, and even less time to actually sit down and eat. Exercising makes our time even tighter and quality nutrition even more crucial. Wouldn't some convenient and nutritious choices make life a lot easier?

At last! Here come the Yummy Hunters to the rescue. What better way than to have a ton of taste-testing palates inform you about scrumptious yet lower calorie appetizers, snacks, sides, entrées and desserts?

The Yummy Hunters serve up oodles of terrific options in tasty categories full of quality nutrition. Every item is categorized with neat details, including availability, calorie content per serving and Yummy notes on taste. Plus, they also single out low-fat foods that are "heart smart." Awesome!

Helen and Eric's charm, knowledge and wit shine through as they share their culinary adventures tasting the yummiest, best-tasting, lower calorie foods.

We live in a world with an endless array of conflicting information pertaining to health, nutrition and food choices. Always consider that eating all foods in moderation plays a key role in healthy weight management and overall wellness.

Proper nutritional intake in conjunction with a quality exercise program can prevent and reduce the risks of chronic conditions. "Your health is your wealth", therefore, food variety and balance become the two main ingredients.

As an elementary concept of nutrition, balance plays a crucial role in energy metabolism. A balanced plan rewards you with stable blood sugars, extended energy, greater mental focus and helps prevent the breakdown of muscle tissue. Additionally, a wide variety of foods keeps your meals interesting.

The important thing is to follow a sensible plan that will gradually help you reach a realistic goal. Start with small and easily obtainable steps to reap the rewards of success!

The Yummy Hunter's Guide is a truly fabulous resource even for the most conscientious and well informed. It's a user-friendly reference tool that can guide you through the maze of supermarket shelves and teach you that eating healthy never means giving up choices. Thanks to this guide, you can be adventurous and expand your tastes. Try something new!

So dive right in and you'll find a delicious blend of delectable "good for you" goodies from soup to nuts. The outcome will be a longer, more vigorous life that's well worth the effort. Thanks, Helen and Eric, for the Yummy details. It's time to eat!

Scott Josephson, M.S.
—Exercise Physiologist and Dietitian Specializing in Weight Achievement
—Contributing Writer for *Fitness Management and Club Life*

INTRODUCTION
A LITTLE HISTORY

Low-calorie foods, ugh, ah, gag! I'd almost rather eat cardboard. I'd almost rather do a hundred more sit-ups! I'd almost rather be fat! If you're someone who watches your weight, you know what I'm talking about.

I grew up fat, and when I was young, I cursed the food companies who produced such dreadful, low-cal products. In my late teens I realized that to keep to my diet and maintain my weight loss I had better find low-cal products I wanted to eat.

Hi, I'm Helen Brand and I'm a certified personal trainer with over 20 years of experience. I have never stopped looking for delicious, low-cal products, and when I uncover one, I share it with my clients. These products quickly find their way into their diet plans and make their dieting more enjoyable and thus more successful.

Two years ago, one of my clients brought in a bag of cookies. "Helen," she squealed in delight, "you must taste this!" I thought, Oh, God, the last thing I want is for others in the gym to get a whiff of these wonderfully aromatic and, to my mind, highly caloric cookies. "No calories, no calories," she repeated over and over, as if caught up in a religious trance.

I took a bite and a warm, satisfying wave of sweet, delightful flavors rushed through my body. I grabbed the bag and studied the contents. There it was, in black and white: 0 calories.

How could I have missed this incredible find? The answer was simple. My client purchased these cookies while visiting relatives. Meanwhile, a group of clients gathered around and begged me to find the cookies locally. While I was at it, they suggested, perhaps I could type up the list of all my discoveries so they could have it when they went food shopping.

Someone suggested I turn it into a book, and suddenly I was inspired. I contacted my writing partner, Eric Robespierre. Eric's a former advertising copywriter who never had to worry about his weight until middle age, when a bulge suddenly appeared above his belt line.

Eric immediately saw the book's benefits and potential for helping dieters all over the country. It was then *The Yummy Hunter's Guide* was conceived and the Yummy Hunters group formed.

What's a Yummy Hunter?

Eric and I realized we couldn't find all the foods on our own. We needed people from all over the country if we were to succeed in creating a comprehensive guide. Because our mission was to discover low-cal foods that taste yummy, we called them Yummy Hunters. We began by asking clients, family members and friends to join the hunt. The response was overwhelming. This first group of Yummy Hunters enlisted a second group, and the circle grew larger and larger.

Yummy Hunters are dieters just like you. They are constantly battling weight problems; going on and off, on and off one diet after another. And, like you, they search supermarket shelves, walk the aisles of health food stores and explore Internet sites looking, buying, trying low-cal foods in the hope of finding the salad dressing that knocks their socks off, the prepared meal that doesn't taste prepared, the chips they can dip without breaking the calorie bank.

Yummy Hunter reviews are straightforward and personal.

What's So Special About Helen and Eric?

Other than coming up with the idea, we are just an average Jane and Joe like our Yummy Hunters and like you. We do not have sophisticated palates, nor do we have any particular gifts that make us connoisseurs of taste. Our comments are solely subjective and never influenced by outside factors except an unhealthy addiction to chocolate.

We get a Yummy Hunter recommendation and then we taste the product for ourselves. Sometimes we agree with the Yummy Hunter, sometimes we disagree. There are times when we exclude a product. When that happens, it's because of the following reasons:

1. The product can't be purchased throughout the United States. We define *purchased throughout the United States* to mean at a retail store, by mail, by phone or over the Internet.

2. It isn't low in calories. We define *low in calories* by comparing it to other products in a category; if it contains more calories than similar products, it doesn't meet our low-cal criterion.

3. There are other products in the same category our Yummy Hunters like better.

4. We can't stand the taste. We define *can't stand the taste* to mean our faces contort into ugly positions, our eyes bulge out of their sockets and we spit the food into the sink.

We might add, sometimes Eric or I discover the product and, in those cases, we become the Yummy Hunter.

What You're Going to Get from This Book

For those of you who never thought there was such a thing as a delicious low-calorie food, you're in for a treat. For those of you who knew such foods existed, but were frustrated because you had to buy six bottles of dressing to find the one that tasted just OK, your salad days are just beginning!

There are over 670 foods in 43 different categories. Yummy Hunters provide reviews of their submissions. Then Eric and I add our own reviews. These product reviews take the guesswork out of shopping for you. They will give you important insights into each food and will help you determine if the product is something you want to try for yourself and your family.

This translates into saving time and money and pays off with delicious-tasting, low-cal products that make your dieting more enjoyable and ultimately more successful.

How the Book Is Arranged

There are 43 categories, some of which have subcategories. Within each category, foods are arranged in alphabetical order by flavor or, in some instances, by product type.

Under each food item is manufacturer/distributor contact information. This is followed by the Bottom Line, denoting calories per serving. Caloric and serving size information comes right from the product labeling and our own inquiries. This is followed by details comprising the Yummy Hunter reviews and then our own remarks. Last comes availability information, which describes all the ways you may purchase the product.

Keep in mind, everything is subjective. Yes, *wowee* is a real word! Remember, we told you these folks are just like you, so there won't be any highfalutin explanations! We do edit Yummy Hunter reviews for clarity and brevity.

Will You Agree with Our Choices?

What's that saying, a couple hundred Yummy Hunters can't be wrong? Seriously, we hope the selected foods make your taste buds tingle, but only time will tell, so please let us know your thoughts by e-mail or through regular mail.

Where Do Low-Fat Foods Fit In?

A new diet plan seems to pop up each year, and the current trend is low fat. To accommodate this movement, we place an asterisk next to all our low-fat food entries. We define a low-fat food as one in which the total amount of fat is 5 grams or less per serving.

We are not here to tell you which diet to follow, only to make the experience of dieting more fulfilling and more enjoyable.

Will This Book Make Your Dieting More Successful?

The foods in *The Yummy Hunter's Guide* can be incorporated into your own weight-loss management program, so whichever diet plan you've chosen, you are assured these foods will smoothly integrate into your daily way of life and help you achieve lifelong success.

Our Yummy Hunters discovered foods that renewed and reenergized their diet plans and drove away the boredom that led them to overeat.

The Yummy Hunter's Guide makes finding mouth-watering low-cal foods simple and easy. Use it to make your shopping list, or carry it with you and refer to it when making an unplanned stop at your local supermarket or health food store. Now, thanks to *The Yummy Hunter's Guide*, you won't have to waste time and money shopping for things you don't like, a process that threatens your sanity and could destroy any diet regime. *The Yummy Hunter's Guide* educates and helps you effectively manage calorie counts, serving sizes and portion-control issues.

Our Bottom Line gives you the calories per serving as stated on the package or manufacturer's website. In our reviews we alert you when one of our choices may be a little high in calories compared with other products in that category, and we tell you the reasons the product has nevertheless been selected.

So, now you are aware of the calorie count, but when you dole out the serving size, you say to yourself, This isn't a serving, this is just my first bite! *The Yummy Hunter's Guide* takes this into consideration and warns you about exceeding the serving size.

This brings us to portion control, the bane of all dieters' existence.

Let's face it, certain foods trigger our emotions. Suddenly our math and reasoning skills disappear. Calorie counts and serving sizes go out the window. I've met people, and you may be one, who cannot stop at one cookie. If I'm at a party and I see a bowl of M&M's, I make sure all my conversations are within an arm's reach of that bowl.

Our reviews make constant reference to portion control and to the foods that trigger our emotions. These references will alert you to your own trigger foods. Portion control is particularly important when dealing with the foods in this book because these foods are so delicious, your natural inclination will be to eat more than the serving size. Eric and I can testify to that.

Oh, a trick I've learned to avoid those M&M's: I bring the host low-calorie sweets as a gift so I know that she'll put out something that I can enjoy without going off my diet!

A Word from Eric

This project came at the perfect time in my life. Like so many middle-aged American males, I'm suddenly saddled with a sluggish metabolism and extra inches I would like to hack off with a meat cleaver. I've been thin all my life. Watching what I ate and counting calories were for other people. You can imagine how unprepared I was when, suddenly, I had a weight problem. I skipped meals, cut down on bread and pasta. I didn't have a plan, so nothing was accomplished. Then I began working with Helen on this book. Now, instead of being a lost soul in the supermarket, I'm an explorer armed with a road map to a better way to eat. I'm full of hope, knowing that at any moment I could discover a great-tasting, low-calorie food that will satisfy my hunger and be perfect for my diet plan.

Final Thoughts

In our reviews we try to inject a little humor. It's not because we don't take the subject matter seriously. We know being overweight can lead to severe heath problems. It's precisely because the subject is so serious that we feel we want to make you smile and even laugh and, in doing so, bring you some emotional satisfaction. Maybe the battle will then be a little easier and the process of weight management a lot more enjoyable. That is also the reason we put humorous quips at the end of each category. These come from Helen and from anonymous authors submitted over the Internet.

Become a Yummy Hunter

The 2006 edition of *The Yummy Hunter's Guide* is our second edition! We intend to continue publishing revised and even more comprehensive guides annually. To help us achieve this goal, we invite you to become a Yummy Hunter. Simply go to www.yummyhunters.com and fill out a Yummy Hunters form or mail us your recommendations at Romax Publishing, P.O. Box 2290, Halesite, NY 11743. We welcome all comments, funny and otherwise!

One last thing, before you go on any diet, consult your physician.

Eat smart, eat well and be happy!

— *Helen and Eric*

HOW TO USE THIS BOOK

The Yummy Hunter's Guide provides you with a list of a vast array of mouth-watering, low-cal products and makes it a snap for you to select and then purchase them quickly and easily.

You will discover more than 670 delicious products in 43 food categories. Simply go to the table of contents to find an alphabetized list of categories. Then go to the selected category to find an alphabetized list, by flavor, of all products.

For those of you who love to use an index, go to the back of the book and you'll find two: a company and product index as well as a food index.

There are certain foods we call crossovers; for instance, Stuffed Chicken Breasts with Broccoli and Cheese can be found in Poultry as well as Meals.

Under each category, we list each product's flavor first; yes "Alphabet" is a flavor, folks! Then we put the product name, and then contact information. We include the manufacturer's name in front of the product name when we think it will help you find the product more quickly.

We include the manufacturer contact information because we thought you might want to contact the manufacturer/distributor. Do not hold back on your praise or your criticism—manufacturers/ distributors do listen to their customers!

Now that we've described what each category lists, here's the way we've designed each entry:

Bottom Line: Only interested in the calories — go to the Bottom Line and rejoice!

Details: This is where you'll find the Yummy Hunter reviews and our own personal comments: Yummy Hunters are the people responsible for finding the products in the book. Their reviews turned us on to the foods. We hope the reviews do the same for you. Yummy Hunters are people like you. Their comments are honest, down-to-earth and from the heart. We edit all Yummy Hunter reviews for clarity and brevity. In some cases we discover the product and so become the Yummy Hunter.

Availability: *The Yummy Hunter's Guide* lists only foods you can buy nationwide and/or by phone or over the Internet.

✷ This asterisk designates a low-fat product. Our definition of a low-fat product is one in which the total amount of fat is 5 grams or less per serving.

ACKNOWLEDGMENTS

WE WOULD LIKE TO THANK all our Yummy Hunters who have contributed their discoveries, nifty quotes and words of inspiration. Our Yummy Hunters are indeed the heart, the soul and the taste buds of this book.

We thank Craig Lowy, our talented designer, who most creatively and meticulously turned our manuscript into a professional-looking book. His unwavering dedication and expertise in so many areas, combined with his wonderful sense of humor, made every moment working with him an absolute pleasure.

Hats off to Julie Shea, who opened our eyes and ultimately our heads when she came up with the "exploding foods" concept for the cover and ultimately extended it out when she designed our website.

Thanks to our proofreaders Dan Young and Christina Palaia and our indexer Michelle Graye, who provided their invaluable expertise and support.

We wish to express our gratitude to Lori and Lenny DeCostanzo, for without their support this book would not have come to fruition.

Last, we would like to thank our families and friends for their love, their encouragement and their willingness to taste whatever foods we shoved in front of them.

DEDICATION

In loving memory of

Maxwell Robespierre

August 7, 1916 – September 8, 2003

THE
YUMMY
HUNTER'S
GUIDE

THE BEST-TASTING

LOW-CALORIE FOODS

AND

WHERE TO SHOP FOR THEM

2006

APPETIZERS

IF THE WORD *appetizer* comes from appetite, how come they're always so small when our appetites are big? Anyway, they've come a long way. Many times a selection of appetizers makes for a very satisfying meal; on other occasions they set up the dinner. In any event, keep to the portion size or else these little starters will be the ends to your dieting plan.

✳ Broccoli and Cheddar
Health Is Wealth, Broccoli Munchees
Val Vasilef, Health Is Wealth Products, Inc.
856-728-1998 www.healthiswealthfoods.com
Bottom Line: 60 calories per serving (2 munchees)
Details: Yummy Hunters think they're nice and thick and like the fact the liquid cheese doesn't fall onto their chins. *Helen:* A delicious, whole-wheat flavor on the outside and just the right amount of tasty cheese and broccoli on the inside. *Eric:* From one sloppy Yummy Hunter to another, I hear ya.
Availability: Supermarkets and health food stores

Buffalo
Morning Star Farms, Buffalo Wings
Kelloggs Co.
800-557-6525 www.morningstarfarms.com
Bottom Line: 200 calories per serving (5 wings)
Details: Yummy Hunters say these wings taste like the real thing, even fooling their husbands, who gobbled them up. *Helen:* Anything that keeps a marriage together gets an A in my book. *Eric:* These wings have a kick to them that'll make your taste buds fly high.
Availability: Supermarkets

✳ Cheese
Empire, Cheese Blintzes
Empire Kosher Poultry, Inc.
800-367-4734 www.empirekosher.com
Bottom Line: 90 calories per serving (1 blintz)
Details: Yummy Hunters recommend them because
they taste delicious and are so simple to make.
They bake them using Pam spray on a cookie sheet,
and the blintzes come out crispy. *Helen:* We ate
them with lite sour cream on top. I needed two to
make my morning, but Eric is a fool for these
beauties and three was his magic number. *Eric:* I
stand convicted.
Availability: Supermarkets in the kosher foods
section and online at www.mykoshermarket.com

✳ Chicken
Health Is Wealth, Chicken-Free Fingers
Val Vasilef, Health Is Wealth Products, Inc.
856-728-1998 www.healthiswealthfoods.com
Bottom Line: 70 calories per serving (2 oz)
Details: Our Yummy Hunters say these nuggets are
low-cal, healthy and delectable. They taste like
the real thing. *Helen:* We agree with our Yummy
Hunters. We couldn't tell these appetizing nuggets
were chicken-free. Crunchy on the outside and
tender on the inside. *Eric:* I dipped mine in honey
mustard sauce and they had me clucking for joy.
Yum yum!
Availability: Supermarkets and health food stores

Chicken
T.G.I. Friday's, Sweet & Smoky Popcorn Chicken
H.J. Heinz Company
800-457-9810 www.fridays.com
Bottom Line: 160 calories per serving (3 pieces)
Details: Yummy Hunters who enjoy Popcorn Chicken
at T.G.I. Friday's are glad they can now have them
at home. They eat six pieces and it makes for a
very special dinner. *Helen & Eric:* Great to eat on
Friday, or any day of the week. These fancy little
nuggets cook up crunchy and don't disappoint.
Availability: Supermarkets

Eggplant
Alessi, Eggplant Appetizer
Vigo Importing Co., Inc.
www.vigoalessi.com
Bottom Line: 140 calories per serving (⅓ cup)
Details: Yummy Hunters say they serve this appetizer to their picky Italian in-laws, who think it's homemade. Others add they like the authentic, delicious taste. *Helen:* We love it on pumpernickel with chopped onions and applaud Alessi for providing products with an authentic taste. *Eric:* I'm still clapping . . . and eating.
Availability: Supermarkets

Hummus with Vegetables
Wakim's Hummus with Vegetables
Wakim's Food, Inc.
215-758-3420
Bottom Line: 50 calories per serving (2 tbsp)
Details: Yummy Hunters love this Middle Eastern delicacy that adds exotic flavor and livens up their normal food plan. *Helen:* This Middle Eastern dish made of chick peas, veggies and interesting seasonings is quickly catching the fancy of Yummy Hunters across the United States, and I can see why. *Eric:* It's really delicious. Slice up some pita bread and have a ball!
Availability: Supermarkets and health food stores

* Mozzarella
Health Is Wealth, Mozzarella Sticks
Val Vasilef, Health Is Wealth Products, Inc.
856-728-1998 www.healthiswealthfoods.com
Bottom Line: 120 calories per serving (2 sticks)
Details: Yummy Hunters who love mozzarella sticks can once again enjoy them while dieting. Others say these are as good as they get in any restaurant. *Helen:* Everything a good mozzarella stick should be and more. We dunked them in Prego's Traditional Pasta Sauce and they were delicious. *Eric:* Crunchy on the outside, soft and gooey on the inside. These sticks stick out.
Availability: Supermarkets and health food stores

* Sesame Peanut
White Wave, Baked Tofu, Thai Style
White Wave, Inc.
www.whitewave.com
Bottom Line: 90 calories per serving (¼ pckg)
Details: Yummy Hunters who are vegetarians and eat lots of tofu tell us this baked Thai flavor is so good they slice it and eat it plain. *Helen:* We sliced it and ate it on Melba toast with a few sprouts on top and it was wondrously delicious. *Eric:* Even if you've never tried tofu, or you have and you hate it, this exotic flavoring makes this a must-try.
Availability: Supermarkets, health food stores; store locations online

* Spinach Artichoke
Classy Delites, Spinach Artichoke Dip
Classy Delites, Inc.
800-440-2648   www.classydelites.com
Bottom Line: 20 calories per serving (2 tbsp)
Details: Yummy Hunters are always happy when they can find a unique-tasting, low-fat dip that keeps them from living in dieting boredom. They say this is a hit with company. *Helen:* This is great stuff. Cut up veggies and have some fun. *Eric:* I say, eat it right off of the spoon—a very big spoon.
Availability: Supermarkets, gourmet shops and ordering online

* Thai
Health Is Wealth, Spring Rolls
Val Vasilef, Health Is Wealth Products, Inc.
856-728-1998   www.healthiswealthfoods.com
Bottom Line: 90 calories per serving (2 pieces)
Details: Yummy Hunters say it's foods like this that keep them on their diets. Others add they make for a unique and tasty meal, anytime of the day. *Helen:* Spicy, crunchy and delicious. I'm always afraid to order one in a restaurant because of the unknown calorie count, but with this product I know I'm getting exactly 90 calories. *Eric:* It's as good as anything I've had in any Thai restaurant.
Availability: Supermarkets and health food stores

* A Low-Fat Product

* Thai
Health Is Wealth, Thai Munchees
Val Vasilef, Health Is Wealth Products, Inc.
856-728-1998 www.healthiswealthfoods.com
Bottom Line: 180 calories per serving (85 g)
Details: Yummy Hunters love the savory spice of this delicious appetizer. *Helen:* Another ethnic food that is delighting our Yummy Hunters and making dieting delicious. *Eric:* As good I get when I order in, makes for a great appetizer or just something to munch on during the day.
Availability: Supermarkets and health food stores

Turkey
Rosina, Italian Style Turkey Meatballs
Rosina Food Products, Inc.
888-767-4621 www.rosina.com
Bottom Line: 170 calories per serving (3 meatballs)
Details: Yummy Hunters declare they've given up homemade meatballs because of this tasty and convenient product. Other dieters, who know how difficult it is to regulate the making of meatballs, are thrilled that this product puts an end to that problem. *Helen & Eric:* We think they're the most delicious store-bought meatballs we've ever eaten, turkey or otherwise.
Availability: Supermarkets

Vegetable
Alexian, Vegetable Pâté
Alexian
800-927-9473 www.alexianpate.com
Bottom Line: 45 calories per serving (2 oz)
Details: Yummy Hunters say they feel like a fine chef when they serve this to their families. They are amazed at how such a gourmet food can be so low in calories. *Helen:* Great on crackers and pumpernickel bread.I suggest you watch the portion size. This product is higher in fat than other appetizers. *Eric:* A delicious aftertaste will have you licking your lips after eating this wonderful pâté.
Availability: Gourmet shops and health food stores

✱ Veggie
Health Is Wealth, Veggie Egg Rolls
Val Vasilef, Health Is Wealth Products, Inc.
856-728-1998 www.healthiswealthfoods.com
Bottom Line: 130 calories per serving (1 roll)
Details: Yummy Hunters rave about how much they love these veggie egg rolls and tell us they're right up there with those from the local Chinese restaurant. *Helen & Eric:* Two rolls are a real meal, but one is great for a snack.
Availability: Supermarkets and health food stores

✱ Veggie
Veggie Patch, Veggie Meatballs
Veggie Patch Products
888-698-3444 www.veggiepatch.com
Bottom Line: 130 calories per serving (4 meatballs)
Details: Yummy Hunters talk about bringing up their kids to be vegetarians and how these low-cal meatballs have become a staple in their households. They love finding unique toppings that make these meatballs special to them. *Helen & Eric:* Reminds us of a falafel with its tantalizing combination of fresh ingredients.
Availability: Supermarkets, health food stores, Wal-Mart and store locations online

Amazing! You hang something in your closet for a while and it shrinks two sizes.

BARS

Without question, bars are the *El Supremo* of snack foods. How we choose our snacks determines how we choose our meals. If the snack is tasty, filling and nourishing, everything else falls into place. But be "bar-ware": All bars are not created equal. Some bars are for snacking, some for meal replacement and others for energy. Watch the calories and choose your bars wisely.

Almond
Nature Valley Sweet & Salty Nut Granola Bars
General Mills, Inc.
800-231-0308 www.naturevalley.com
Bottom Line: 160 calories per serving (1 bar)
Details: Yummy Hunters found this product at a supermarket tasting and said they bought the store out. They add it's the family's number one bar. *Helen:* Thank you, Nature Valley! What women dream about—sweet and salty! *Eric:* I thought women dreamed about making their men happy.
Availability: Supermarkets

* Banana
Humm Foods, Lara Bara, Banana Cookie Bar
Humm Foods
877-527-2227 www.larabar.com
Bottom Line: 210 calories per serving (1 bar)
Details: Yummy Hunters love these bars because they know they're eating something healthy. They add the labeling is clear and concise. *Helen:* Natural fruit taste. High in fiber and made from good stuff. Well worth the extra calories. *Eric:* Chewy, tasty and the banana is not overpowering.
Availability: Health food stores and online

Caramel 'n Chocolate
Balance Nutrition Energy Bar, Carb Well, Caramel 'n Chocolate
Balance Bar Company
800-678-4248 www.balance.com
Bottom Line: 190 calories per serving (1 bar)
Details: Yummy Hunters who love gooey, chocolatey treats are crazy for this bar. *Helen:* Barware! This bar is a little high in calories and fat. Enjoy cautiously. *Eric:* We took a walk on the wild side and froze the bar so we could cut it into smaller pieces, thus making it last longer.
Availability: Health food stores and some supermarkets

* Chocolate
Kraft, South Beach Diet, High Protein Cereal Bars
Kraft Foods North America, Inc.
800-932-7800 www.krafthealthyliving.com
Bottom Line: 140 calories per serving (1 bar)
Details: Yummy Hunters say it is an energizing combo. They add low calorie and low carb make it a terrific choice. *Helen:* Kraft's new South Beach line of protein bars is extremely filling, plus they have a great chocolate taste. And you know what a nut I am for chocolate. *Eric:* You're not the only one. Yum, yum.
Availability: Supermarkets

* Chocolate Caramel Karma
Kashi, Go Lean, Chocolate Caramel Karma
Kashi Company
858-274-8870 www.kashi.com
Bottom Line: 140 calories per serving (1 bar)
Details: Yummy Hunters exclaim—what a great combo! They love the chocolate, the rich caramel and the great crunch. *Helen:* It's a whale of a bar for the 140 calories. We love chocolate and caramel, so imagine getting two bangs for the bite! *Eric:* I believe it's my karma to enjoy this chocolate caramel treat.
Availability: Supermarkets, health food stores and online

* A Low-Fat Product

✳ Chocolate Chip Cookie Dough
Glenny's, Light N Crispy, Chocolate Chip Cookie Dough
Glen Foods, Inc.
888-864-1243 www.glennys.com
Bottom Line: 70 calories per serving (1 bar)
Details: Yummy Hunters love to share these cookie dough treats with their kids. *Helen & Eric:* Cookie dough makes us feel like kids, too!
Availability: Health food stores and some supermarkets; store locations and ordering online

✳ Chocolate Crisp
Just 2 Points, Nutritional Snack Bar, Chocolate Crisp
Weight Watchers International, Inc.
800-815-8704 www.weightwatchers.com
Bottom Line: 100 calories per serving (1 bar)
Details: Yummy Hunters love the rich, chocolatey flavor. *Helen & Eric*: Great crunch, too.
Availability: Weight Watchers Meeting Centers

✳ Chocolate Peanut Butter
Apex Fix Crisp Chocolate Peanut Butter Bar
Apex Fitness Group
800-656-2739 www.apexfitness.com
Bottom Line: 160 calories per serving (1 bar)
Details: One starving Yummy Hunter, after her morning workout, ate a bar and could not believe this kept her satisfied until dinner. *Helen & Eric:* We loved the crispy, light chocolate covering and the fact that it only has 4 grams of fat.
Availability: Ordering online and in some gyms

Chocolate Raspberry Fudge
Balance, Chocolate Raspberry Fudge
Balance Bar Company
800-678-4248. www.balance.com
Bottom Line: 200 calories per serving (1 bar)
Details: Yummy Hunters say when they can't get out for lunch this bar saves the day. *Helen & Eric:* Tastes like chocolate-covered raspberries. Truth be told, we might skip lunch just to have one.
Availability: Health food stores and some supermarkets

✱ Cinnamon
Quaker, Oatmeal Breakfast Squares, Brown Sugar Cinnamon
Quaker Oats Company
800-856-5781 www.quakeroats.com
Bottom Line: 220 calories per serving (1 bar)
Details: Yummy Hunters tell us they grew up eating sweets with breakfast and, although donuts were their favorites, these squares are now all they eat. *Helen:* So, when it comes to sweets—to avoid getting round, look for a square. *Eric:* I love it when Helen gets geometrical.
Availability: Supermarkets

✱ Cinnamon Raisin
Nutri Snack Cinnamon Raisin Bar
Nutritious Creations, LTD
631-666-9815 www.bakedgoods.tv
Bottom Line: 164 calories per serving (3 oz)
Details: One Yummy Hunter told us this is one quick and easy breakfast that satisfies her sweet tooth. *Helen:* I encourage Yummy Hunters not to make a practice of this and to eat a balanced breakfast whenever they can. *Eric:* The perfect blend of cinnamon and raisin with a chewy consistency that makes this a true winner.
Availability: Some health food stores, delis and online

✱ Coffee Chocolate Chip
Glenny's, Light N Crispy Coffee Chocolate Chip
Glen Foods, Inc.
888-864-1243 www.glennys.com
Bottom Line: 60 calories per serving (1 bar)
Details: Yummy Hunters love the crunchiness of this bar. Another adds it's only 1 point on Weight Watchers. *Helen:* A subtle coffee flavor with a rich chocolatey taste makes this one heavenly 60-calorie treat. *Eric:* This is one great between-meal snack! Coffee lovers—you'll love it.
Availability: Health food stores and some supermarkets; store locations and ordering online

Cookies'N Caramel
Pria, Carb Select Bar Cookies'N Caramel
PowerBar, Inc.
800-587-6937 www.powerbar.com
Bottom Line: 170 calories per serving (1 bar)
Details: Yummy Hunters say it's hard to find a great-tasting, low-carb bar, but this one fits the bill. *Helen & Eric:* None of the soy taste you usually find in low-carb bars, just plenty of cookies and caramel! What a joy!
Availability: Supermarkets, health food stores, wholesale clubs and gourmet shops; store locations and ordering online

Cranberry Almond
Quaker, Q-Smart, Cranberry Almond
Quaker Oats Company
800-856-5781 www.quakeroats.com
Bottom Line: 120 calories per serving (1 bar)
Details: Yummy Hunters know that eating nuts can put them on the road to disaster, but this fruit and nut combo satisfies the urge and at the same time keeps them out of trouble. *Helen:* The cranberries pack a nice wallop. I love dry fruit and nuts, too, but I can lose control, so this bar is a winner with me. *Eric:* Despite what Helen might say, when it comes to nuts, I am always in complete control. *Helen:* Not!
Availability: Supermarkets

* Date
Health Valley, Date Bakes
Hain Celestial Group, Inc.
800-434-4246 www.hain-celestial.com
Bottom Line: 70 calories per serving (1 bar)
Details: Yummy Hunters like the great combination of flavors and say it's something the entire family loves. *Helen:* When you're counting calories, this bar is the right snack choice. Subtle but delicious fruity taste. *Eric:* You've got to make a date with this bar.
Availability: Supermarkets, health food stores and ordering online at www.naturemart.com

* Fudge Dip Soy Bar
Glenny's, Light N Crispy, Fudge Dip Soy Bar
Glen Foods, Inc.
888-864-1243 www.glennys.com
Bottom Line: 60 calories per serving (1 bar)
Details: One Yummy Hunter jumped for joy over this 1-point Weight Watcher's wonder. *Helen:* A crunchy, great fudge-flavored soy bar! *Eric:* I dip my hat to Glenny's!
Availability: Health food stores and some supermarkets; store locations and ordering online

* Granola Nut
Starbucks Penza, Granola Nut Bar
Manufacturer for Starbucks Coffee Company
800-235-2883 www.starbucks.com
Bottom Line: 170 calories per serving (1 bar)
Details: Yummy Hunters tell us they love their Starbucks coffee in the afternoon. They add when ordering latte with low-fat milk, they had a problem resisting the pastries until they discovered this granola bar. This was just the thrill they needed. *Helen:* We just came back from Starbucks and all we can say is the thrill's on us! *Eric:* This was some grande, granola, nut bar.
Availability: Starbucks

* Lemon-Lime
Kashi, Go Lean, Go Lean, Crunchy! Bar, Sublime Lemon-Lime
Kashi Company
858-274-8870 www.kashi.com
Bottom Line: 160 calories per serving (1 bar)
Details: Yummy Hunters say when they're dieting they are always searching for a new taste and this is a home run for them and their families. *Helen:* This unique flavor can refresh anyone's diet. Sweet and satisfying. *Eric:* A great new product. This intriguing combo of lemon-lime makes for a sublime treat. Go lean, go lime, go Kashi.
Availability: Supermarkets, health food stores and online

* Marshmallow
Kellogg's, Rice Krispies Treats, Marshmallow
Kellogg Co.
800-962-1516 www.kelloggs.com
Bottom Line: 90 calories per serving (1 bar)
Details: One Yummy Hunter says she took them out of the wrapper, put them on a dish and her kids actually thought she made these delicious treats by herself. *Helen:* They remind me of the after-school treats my mom made me. *Eric:* Some kids have all the luck.
Availability: Supermarkets

* Mint Chocolate
Pria, Mint Chocolate Cookie Flavor
PowerBar, Inc.
800-587-6937 www.powerbar.com
Bottom Line: 110 calories per serving (1 bar)
Details: One Yummy Hunter told us she and her husband split one for their after-dinner treat and it reminded them of the mints they get at their favorite, fancy restaurant. *Helen:* I like to have something sweet after lunch and dinner. This refreshing mint bar kept me from reaching for a more fattening dessert. *Eric:* I smacked my lips and said, "Girl Scout cookies. Yeah!"
Availability: Supermarkets, health food stores, wholesale clubs and gourmet shops; store locations, ordering online and at www.performancebike.com

Nutty S'Mores
Skippy, Trail Mix
Unilever
800-866-4skippy
Bottom Line: 150 calories per serving (1 bar)
Details: Yummy Hunters say they love this gooey, chewy trail mix bar. *Helen:* Baby marshmallows, tasty chocolate chips and lots of peanuts make this one fabulous bar. *Eric:* What a happy combo. This bar will have you singing "Happy Trails to You!"
Availability: Supermarkets

✳ Oatmeal Raisin
Just 2 Points, Nutritional Snack Bar, Chewy Oatmeal Raisin
Weight Watchers International, Inc.
800-815-8704 www.weightwatchers.com
Bottom Line: 140 calories per serving (1 bar)
Details: Yummy Hunters say the raisins make this oatmeal bar a heavenly breakfast. *Helen & Eric:* Light but not too sweet.
Availability: Weight Watchers Meeting Centers; center locations online

✳ Orange
NuGo Nutrition To Go, Orange Smoothie
NuGo Nutrition
888-421-2032 www.nugonutrition.com
Bottom Line: 190 calories per serving (1 bar)
Details: Yummy Hunters rave creamsicle taste in a bar. Hurray! *Helen:* Perfect combo, perfect bar. *Eric:* Great taste of orange in a protein bar. This smoothie is real smooth!
Availability: Limited supermarkets and health food stores; store locations and ordering online

✳ Peanut Butter
Post, Carb Well, Peanut Butter
Kraft Foods, North America
800-431-7678 www.kraftfoods.com
Bottom Line: 140 calories per serving (1 bar)
Details: Yummy Hunters enjoy the way this crunchy peanut cereal bar keeps them full between meals. They keep one in their desk drawers for that famine emergency. *Helen:* Crunchy with peanuts throughout and peanut butter frosting on top. Believe me, it tastes just as good as it sounds. *Eric:* Peanut butter overwhelms, just the way I like it.
Availability: Supermarkets

Peanut Butter
Slim-Fast, Meal Options, Peanut Butter
Slim-Fast Foods Company
877-345-4632 www.slim-fast.com
Bottom Line: 150 calories per serving (1 bar)

Details: One Yummy Hunter tells us if she substitutes this bar for lunch during the week, she is able to splurge a little while dining out with her husband on the weekends. *Helen & Eric:* We love it, but if you're really hungry, we don't think it's filling enough to replace a meal.
Availability: Supermarkets and drugstores

* Peanut Caramel
Just 2 Points, Nutritional Snack Bar, Peanut Caramel
Weight Watchers International, Inc.
800-815-8704 www.weightwatchers.com
Bottom Line: 140 calories per serving (1 bar)
Details: Yummy Hunters rave it's as good as any candy they've ever eaten. They like to slice it and eat one piece at a time. *Helen & Eric:* Awesome!
Availability: Weight Watchers Meeting Centers

* Peanut Caramel
Slim-Fast, Snack Options, Peanut Caramel, Crispy
Slim-Fast Foods Company
877-345-4632 www.slim-fast.com
Bottom Line: 120 calories per serving (1 bar)
Details: Yummy Hunters are irresistibly drawn to the wonderful combination of flavors and say one bar is enough to satisfy their cravings for a chocolate snack. *Helen & Eric:* Great chocolatey, gooey taste, the peanut caramel makes for an extremely satisfying experience.
Availability: Supermarkets and drugstores

* Sesame Raisin
Luna, Sesame Raisin Crunch
Clif Bar, Inc.
800-lunabar www.lunabar.com
Bottom Line: 170 calories per serving (1 bar)
Details: Yummy Hunters say taste wins out over fat, calories and carbs when choosing a bar. *Helen:* I agree and it doesn't do too bad in the other areas, either. *Eric:* Open Sesame and let the raisins in! Yahoo!
Availability: Health food stores; store locations and ordering online and at www.leesmarket.com

* S'mores
Quaker, S'mores, Chewy Granola Bars
Quaker Oats Company
800-856-5781 www.quakeroats.com
Bottom Line: 110 calories per serving (1 bar)
Details: Yummy Hunters say it's like eating s'mores without the guilt. *Helen:* I never thought this incredible combo could fit into anybody's diet. It captures the flavor of that great camping favorite. *Eric:* The only thing that's missing is the campfire and the scary stories.
Availability: Supermarkets

* Strawberry
Kellogg's, Special K Bars, Strawberry
Kellogg Co.
800-962-1516 www.kelloggs.com
Bottom Line: 90 calories per serving (1 bar)
Details: Yummy Hunters love the way the strawberries are blended throughout the bar. They say that when they eat an early breakfast, one bar keeps them going till lunch. *Helen:* I'm a fool for strawberries and I kept eating these sweet treats to see how foolish I could get. *Eric:* The tasty yogurt topping makes our taste buds sing in the key of delicious!
Availability: Supermarkets

* Strawberry
Nature's Choice Multigrain Cereal Bars, Strawberry
Barbara's Bakery, Inc.
707-765-2273 www.barbarasbakery.com
Bottom Line: 120 calories per serving (1 bar)
Details: Yummy Hunters tell us that when they don't have time for breakfast these cereal bars are their first choice. They add that they love the fresh, wholesome and wheaty taste. *Helen:* It's like putting strawberry jam on a piece of multigrain bread. Loved the convenience. Delish! *Eric:* We like to soak 'em in Skim Plus and then eat 'em! Nature's Choice is our choice. Yum, yum!
Availability: Health food stores, some supermarkets and store locations online

* Strawberry
Tropicana Fruit Integrity, Strawberry Fruit Bars
Integrated Brands, Inc.
800-423-2763 www.coolbrandsinternational.com
Bottom Line: 140 calories per serving (1 bar)
Details: Yummy Hunters say it's like fresh fruit jumping out of a bar. Others say it's their kids' favorite. *Helen:* This is one very sweet bar with fruity, strawberry flavor in every bite. *Eric:* I didn't see any jumping fruit, but then again my eyes were closed as I savored every sweet morsel.
Availability: Supermarkets

* Strawberry Cheesecake
Kellogg's, Nutri Grain Twists, Cereal Bars, Strawberry Cheesecake
Kellogg Co.
800-962-1516 www.kelloggs.com
Bottom Line: 140 calories per serving (1 bar)
Details: Yummy Hunters delight in the fact there's the taste of strawberries and cheesecake in every bite. *Helen:* I microwaved one for 20 seconds and it softened enough to eat with a fork. Wonder of wonders! Another taboo product we can enjoy. *Eric:* What a great twist. It's strawberry cheesecake to go!
Availability: Supermarkets

* Strawberry Cobbler
Health Valley, Cereal Bars, Strawberry Cobbler
Health Valley
800-434-4246 www.hain-celestial.com
Bottom Line: 130 calories per serving (1 bar)
Details: One Yummy Hunter reveals that her grandma used to bake strawberry bars when she was a kid, so these rekindle that warm, fuzzy feeling. *Helen:* My grandmother only knew how to make reservations. A strawberry taste sensation. *Eric:* How does that song go — "Strawberry cobblers forever"?
Availability: Supermarkets and ordering online at www.leesmarket.com

✳ Strawberry Yogurt
Puffins, Cereal & Milk Bars, Strawberry Yogurt
Barbara's Bakery, Inc.
707-765-2273 www.barbarasbakery.com
Bottom Line: 130 calories per serving (1 bar)
Details: Yummy Hunters say they have a French-toast-morning flavor. *Helen:* A unique topping complements the richness of the bar. *Eric:* I like to lick the icing off the top and slowly work my way through the rest.
Availability: Supermarkets, health food stores; store locations online

✳ Sweet Dreams
Luna, Sweet Dreams
Clif Bar, Inc.
800-lunabar www.lunabar.com
Bottom Line: 180 calories per serving (1 bar)
Details: Yummy Hunters declare this is a satisfyingly sweet-tasting bar for women on the go. *Helen & Eric:* It has a unique, crunchy, chocolatey topping combined with a tasty undercoat. We applaud the fact they're active sponsors of the Breast Cancer Fund.
Availability: Health food stores; store locations and ordering online and at www.leesmarket.com

✳ Trail Mix
Kashi, Chewy Cranola Bar, Trail Mix
Kashi Company
858-274-8870 www.kashi.com
Bottom Line: 130 calories per serving (1 bar)
Details: Yummy Hunters say this is their "bar on the run." *Helen:* I'll run with that! *Eric:* I prefer a fast-paced walk.
Availability: Supermarkets, health food stores and online

You are what you eat. I'm a chocolate bar!

✳ A Low-Fat Product

BEVERAGES – COLD

COFFEE, JUICE, MILK, SHAKES, SMOOTHIES, SODA, TEA, WATER

Nothing quenches our thirst like a cold beverage, but who wants to drink up calories when we can eat them? Our Yummy Hunters have found the perfect solution and selected a variety of tasty, low-cal blends and brews guaranteed to cool you down and hopefully keep your weight down, too.

COFFEE

* Caramel
Nescafe, Frothé, Captivating Caramel
Nestlé USA, Inc.
800-637-8531 www.nestle.com
Bottom Line: 90 calories per serving (3 tbsp)
Details: Yummy Hunters say this convenient, creamy drink is their first choice when they want something sweet and delicious. *Helen & Eric:* The smooth blend of flavors is as good as any coffeehouse drink.
Availability: Supermarkets

* Chocolate Mocha
Nescafe, Ice Java, Chocolate Mocha
Nestlé USA, Inc.
800-637-8531 www.nestle.com
Bottom Line: 80 calories per serving (2 tbsp)
Details: Yummy Hunters who love chocolate milk rave about this unique product. They tell us it's a sweet way to end a meal. *Helen:* Another product we think is as good as any coffeehouse selection. *Eric:* First it was icing on the cake, now it's icing on the java. What will they think of next?
Availability: Supermarkets

✳ French Vanilla
International Coffees, Cappuccino Coolers, French Vanilla
Maxwell House Coffee Company
800-432-6333 www.gfic.com
Bottom Line: 60 calories per serving (1 packet)
Details: One Yummy Hunter, who is always hungry in the afternoon, tells us a glass of this tasty and delicious drink tides her over until dinner. *Helen:* A cool, vanilla sensation. *Eric:* I love the vanilla fragrance of this coffee. Make a second cup and use it as a room freshener.
Availability: Supermarkets

JUICE

✳ Cranberry
Ocean Spray, Light Cranberry Juice Cocktail
Ocean Spray Cranberries, Inc.
800-662-3263 www.oceanspray.com
Bottom Line: 40 calories per serving (8 fl oz)
Details: Yummy Hunters say it's tangy and refreshing. Some say they even have it with their vodka. *Helen:* If it didn't say "Light" on the label, we wouldn't have been able to tell the difference. *Eric:* We drink this by the gallon, but we lose the vodka.
Availability: Supermarkets, convenience stores, drugstores and Wal-Mart

✳ Fruit Punch
Tropicana, Light, Fruit Punch
PepsiCo.
800-237-7799 www.tropicana.com
Bottom Line: 10 calories per serving (8 fl oz)
Details: Yummy Hunters say it's their new favorite. They drink a glass before dinner and say it fills them up, helping them eat less during the meal. *Helen:* Delightful, refreshingly sweet taste. My kids love it. *Eric:* Nothing lightweight about the delicious taste of this light fruit punch.
Availability: Supermarkets

* Guava Citrus
Minute Maid, Light Guava Citrus
The Coca-Cola Company
800-452-2653 www.minutemaid.com
Bottom Line: 5 calories per serving (8 fl oz)
Details: Yummy Hunters love this refreshing, summertime drink that they bring to the beach. *Helen:* The guava does not overpower but creates a very unique and tasty fruit blend. Exotic, fruity and a real taste of the tropics. *Eric:* Why wait until summer? I think this is such a special drink I serve it to friends instead of liquor at afternoon cocktails. *Helen:* Oh please, no one will come to your house. *Eric:* They will now that they know that I serve this.
Availability: Supermarkets

* Lemonade
Minute Maid, Light Lemonade
The Coca-Cola Company
800-452-2653 www.minutemaid.com
Bottom Line: 15 calories per serving (8 fl oz)
Details: Yummy Hunters say they keep cans of this refreshing drink in their fridge. They add that it's sweet yet tangy and has a real, old-fashioned lemonade taste. *Helen:* We agree. This lemony beverage is a true thirst quencher. *Eric:* Something new, something old, something cold; whatever's your choice, this is the real deal.
Availability: Supermarkets

* Limonada-Limeade
Minute Maid, Light, Limonada-Limeade
The Coca-Cola Company
800-452-2653 www.minutemaid.com
Bottom Line: 15 calories per serving (8 fl oz)
Details: Yummy Hunters tell us they love this unusual and refreshing drink that is very rich in fruit taste. *Helen:* Puts a new twist to lemonade. *Eric:* What a dazzling combo of flavors. You're gonna guzzle this baby down.
Availability: Supermarkets

* Orange
Crystal Light, Sunrise, Classic Orange
Kraft Foods, Inc.
800-431-1002 www.crystallight.com
Bottom Line: 5 calories per serving (8 fl oz)
Details: Yummy Hunters who love orange juice are overjoyed because they can drink as much of this as they want without adding lots of calories. *Helen:* It tastes like orangeade to me. *Eric:* I think it tastes more like a creamsicle.
Availability: Supermarkets

* Orange Carrot
Diet Snapple, Orange Carrot
Snapple Beverage Corp.
www.snapple.com
Bottom Line: 10 calories per serving (8 fl oz)
Details: Yummy Hunters recommend this refreshing blend of flavors. *Helen & Eric:* We love the way the orange and carrot juices work so well together.
Availability: Supermarkets

* Raspberry Lime
V8, Diet Splash, Tropical Blend
Campbell Soup Co.
800-871-0988 www.v8juice.com
Bottom Line: 10 calories per serving (8 fl oz)
Details: Yummy Hunters say it's tangy, sweet and so, so refreshing. *Helen:* A masterful blend of fresh juice favors. *Eric:* This combo makes a delicious splash.
Availability: Supermarkets and online at www.netgrocer.com

* Ruby Red Grapefruit
Crystal Light, Ruby Red Grapefruit
Kraft Foods, Inc.
800-431-1002 www.crystallight.com
Bottom Line: 5 calories per serving (8 fl oz)
Details: Yummy Hunters love the tart flavor and prefer it to soda. *Helen:* Interesting and invigorating. *Eric:* Taste that'll ring your bell.
Availability: Supermarkets and online

✱ Vegetable
V8, 100% Vegetable Juice
Campbell Soup Co.
800-871-0988 www.v8juice.com
Bottom Line: 50 calories per serving (8 fl oz)
Details: Yummy Hunters say this is a great
appetizer and an old-time favorite. *Helen:* We love
the smooth blend of veggies and its distinctive
flavor. If you drink one of these before a meal, it
really curbs your appetite. *Eric:* One tangy, tomato
treat. I love it just as much now as I did when I was
a kid.
Availability: Supermarkets

✱ White Grape Raspberry
Welch's Low Cal, White Grape Raspberry
Welch's
800-340-6870 www.welchs.com
Bottom Line: 15 calories per serving (10 fl oz)
Details: Yummy Hunters love something sweet to
drink at breakfast and this one is a favorite. They
add it doesn't leave an acidy taste like some
juices. Another, who doesn't drink alcohol, pours it
over ice and has it when she and her friends are
having cocktails. *Helen & Eric:* It was the perfect
drink when we ate our Better'N Peanut Butter and
Welch's sugar-free jelly.
Availability: Supermarkets

MILK

✱ Chocolate
8th Continent, Soy Milk, Chocolate
General Mills
800-247-6458 www.8thcontinent.com
Bottom Line: 140 calories per serving (8 fl oz)
Details: Yummy Hunters tell us their families think
it's chocolate milk. *Helen:* Rich, chocolatey flavor.
Eric: I have it with my cereal and drink it straight
up when I'm looking for a chocolate jolt. Be
warned, it's addicting.
Availability: Supermarkets

SHAKES

* Double Fudge
Alba Dairy Shake Mix, Double Fudge
Hains Celestial Group, Inc.
800-434-4246 www.albadrinks.com
Bottom Line: 70 calories per serving (8 fl oz, 1 env)
Details: Yummy Hunters who can't give up chocolate rave about this delicious, frosty shake. *Helen & Eric:* Very chocolatey. We added a little less water and a little more ice than recommended on the package, and our shake was so thick, the straw stood straight up.
Availability: Supermarkets

SMOOTHIES

* Chocolate
Weight Watcher's, Smoothie, Creamy Chocolate
Weight Watchers International
800-815-8704 www.weightwatchers.com
Bottom Line: 10 calories per serving (1 packet)
Details: Yummy Hunters tell us when they just have to have chocolate they make a smoothie either with water or low-fat milk. It fills them up for hours. *Helen:* Thick, creamy and so, so much chocolate. For a different twist try adding Dr. Brown's Diet Cream Soda instead of water or milk. *Eric:* A very groovy smoothie.
Availability: Weight Watchers Meeting Centers

* Strawberry Banana
Light 'n Fit Smoothie, Strawberry Banana
Dannon Company, Inc.
877-326-6668 www.dannon.com
Bottom Line: 70 calories per serving (7 fl oz)
Details: Yummy Hunters think it's creamy and fruity, and for 80 calories it fills them up any time of the day. *Helen:* Thick and Yummy! A taste of the tropics. *Eric:* So thick, you could dive into it and not sink. Makes a great moustache.
Availability: Supermarkets

SODA

* Chocolate

Jeff's Diet Chocolate Soda "Amazing My Egg Cream"
Egg Cream America, Inc.
847-559-2703 www.getcreamed.com
Bottom Line: 20 calories per serving (1 bottle)
Details: Yummy Hunters say when they close their eyes they think they're sipping an egg cream at their local soda shop. *Helen:* I'm more of a shakes person, but Eric loves egg creams and he drank the bottle before I could say, "Don't you want a straw?" *Eric:* I did share my smile with her.
Availability: Supermarkets and online

* Cream

Dr. Brown's, Diet Cream Soda
Canada Dry Bottling Company
www.canadadry.com
Bottom Line: 0 calories per serving (1 can)
Details: Yummy Hunters tell us they love to add a scoop of low-fat vanilla ice cream to this cream soda and make their own ice cream soda. They say it tastes just like an old-fashioned fountain drink. *Helen:* A lighter taste alternative to regular colas. *Eric:* Since childhood, one of my favorite flavors. I'm going to follow the Yummy Hunter's suggestion, only I'm going to see what it tastes like with low-fat caramel ice cream.
Availability: Supermarkets

* Orange

Sunkist, Diet Orange Soda
Canned under the joint authority of Dr. Pepper and 7 Up
866-drinkorange www.sunkistsoda.com
Bottom Line: 0 calories per serving (12 fl oz)
Details: Yummy Hunters who love orange soda are all over this product. They are almost evangelical when it comes to singing its praises. *Helen:* Sweet, orangey flavor. *Eric:* Praise Sunkist and pass the soda. Amen!
Availability: Supermarkets

TEA

✳ Lemonade/Tea
Snapple, Diet, Lemonade Iced Tea
Snapple Beverage Corp.
800-696-5891 www.snapple.com
Bottom Line: 10 calories per serving (8 fl oz)
Details: Yummy Hunters say it's like squeezing fresh lemons into their ice tea . *Helen:* As good as I make it and I make it really good. *Eric:* I second the motion.
Availability: Supermarkets

✳ Mandarin & Mango
Lipton Green Tea To Go With Natural Mandarin & Mango Flavors
Unilever
800-290-5266 www.lipton.com
Bottom Line: 0 calories per serving (8 fl oz prepared)
Details: Yummy Hunters love this thirst-quenching, fruit-flavored tea. *Helen & Eric:* Put one packet of Lipton Green Tea together with eight ounces of water in a sport bottle. Shake and go!
Availability: Supermarkets

✳ Plum-A-Granate
Snapple, Diet Plum-A-Granate, Iced Tea
Snapple Beverage Corp.
800-696-5891 www.snapple.com
Bottom Line: 5 calories per serving (8 fl oz)
Details: Yummy Hunters can't believe the delicious combinations of taste. *Helen:* Neither can we. An energizing blend of fruit and tea. *Eric:* I'm plum crazy about it.
Availability: Supermarkets

WATER

✳ Lemon
Perrier, Lemon
Distributed by Great Waters of France
800-937-2002 www.perrier.com
Bottom Line: 0 calories per serving (8 fl oz)

Details: Yummy Hunters praise the refreshing, lemony taste. *Helen:* We, too, love the lemony flavor and find it extremely thirst-quenching. The fizziness makes it more fun to drink. *Eric:* This delicious-tasting drink makes me bubble over with joy and reminds me of my French ancestry.
Availability: Supermarkets

* Peach
Propel, Fitness Water, Peach
The Gatorade Company
877-377-6735 www.propelwater.com
Bottom Line: 10 calories per serving (8 fl oz)
Details: *Helen:* I discovered this at a recent fitness seminar, and for my taste it's the most delicious and refreshing drink on the market. The subtle blending of water and flavoring is unbelievable. *Eric:* What a product! One sip and you'll be propelled into your local supermarket to buy more. Grape and lemon are two additional delicious flavor choices.
Availability: Supermarkets

* Wild Cherry
Mistic, Sparkling, Wild Cherry
Mistic Brands, Inc.
800-764-7842 www.mistic.com
Bottom Line: 0 calories per serving (8 fl oz)
Details: Yummy Hunters can't believe it has no fat, no calories and no carbs, yet loads of cherry soda taste. They declare it's their one and only beverage. *Helen & Eric:* This drink is unbelievable. A must-have.
Availability: New York area and ordering online at www.gethealthyamerica.com

Eat, drink and be merry, for tomorrow we diet.

BEVERAGES – HOT

Cocoa, Coffee, Tea

Two wonderful things about hot beverages: Their warmth gives comfort and the heat prevents you from guzzling down those unwanted calories.

COCOA

✱ Cocoa
Swiss Miss, Diet Hot Cocoa Mix
ConAgra Foods, Inc.
800-457-6649 www.conagrafoods.com
Bottom Line: 25 calories per serving (1 env)
Details: Yummy Hunters declare it's their favorite drink on a cold day. They love the sweet, sweet taste! *Helen:* It's the treat I give myself after I shovel the snow! *Eric:* I'm a city boy, so it's the drink of choice when I'm looking out the window watching someone else do the hard work.
Availability: Supermarkets

COFFEE

✱ Chocolate Mint
Teeccino, Chocolate Mint, Caffeine Free, Herbal Coffee
Teeccino Caffe, Inc.
800-498-3434 www.teeccino.com
Bottom Line: 15 calories per serving (1 tbsp)
Details: Yummy Hunters say they love the flavor and that it's caffeine free. They add it's like having a treat when they're on a diet. *Helen & Eric:* The mint gives it a refreshing flavor, which is surprising in a hot drink. We also recommend Teeccino's hazelnut for the same amount of calories.
Availability: Health food stores, some supermarkets, by phone and online

* French Vanilla
International Coffees, French Vanilla Cafe
Maxwell House Coffee Company
800-432-6333 www.kraftfoods.com
Bottom Line: 25 calories per serving (1 tbsp)
Details: One Yummy Hunter tells us that ever since her daughter was born she's been on a diet. When her child naps, instead of snacking, she makes a cup of French vanilla, puts her feet up and relaxes. Best of all, she's losing weight. *Helen:* Great news. Rich vanilla flavor makes this hot beverage stand apart. *Eric:* Nice story, nice product. And now I know what to do with my feet while I'm drinking coffee.
Availability: Supermarkets

* Mocha
Caffe D'Oro, Mocha Cappuccino
Caffe D'Oro Enterprises
800-253-9517 www.cafedorocappuccino.com
Bottom Line: 35 calories per serving (2 tsp)
Details: Yummy Hunters declare it tastes like the delicious café mocha they get at Starbucks. *Helen:* One cup and we were hooked. *Eric:* I must confess when Helen's back was turned, I went back and made another for myself. *Helen:* He forgets I'm a mom and I have eyes in the back of my head.
Availability: Online

TEA

* Apricot
Laci Le Beau, Super Dieter's Tea, Apricot
Natrol
800-262-8765 www.lacilebeau.com
Bottom Line: 0 calories per serving (1 bag)
Details: Yummy Hunters say the apricot makes this one sweet tea. *Helen:* Big-flavored tea. First time for me, but won't be the last. *Eric:* New, unique flavor.
Availability: Wal-Mart, drug stores; store locations online and ordering online at www.amazon.com

✴ Black Cherry Berry
Celestial Seasonings, Black Cherry Berry, Natural Herbal Tea
Hain Celestial Group, Inc.
800-351-8175 www.celestialseasonings.com
Bottom Line: 0 calories per serving (1 bag)
Details: Yummy Hunters make it their luncheon favorite. *Helen:* The rich cherry flavor is a favorite in my family. *Eric:* Mandarin Orange Spice and Honey Vanilla Chamomile are two other terrific flavors, but check out the entire product line.
Availability: Supermarkets

✴ Black Tea
Stash Premium English Breakfast Black Tea
Stash Tea Company
www.stashtea.com
Bottom Line: 0 calories per serving (1 bag)
Details: Yummy Hunters like the rich taste of this black tea ,and it helps them curb their appetite between meals. *Helen:* A tasty treat, any time of the day. *Eric:* Strong and full of flavor.
Availability: Health food stores and online

✴ Black Tea, Spiced
Tazo, Decaffeinated, Tazo Chai, Spiced Black Tea
Tazo
800-299-9445 www.tazo.com
Bottom Line: 0 calories per serving (1 bag)
Details: Yummy Hunters say it spices up their afternoon tea break. *Helen & Eric:* Rich and tangy.
Availability: Supermarkets

✴ Chocolatte
Guayaki Yerba Mate
Guayaki Sustainable Rainforest Products, Inc.
www.guayaki.com
Bottom Line: 0 calories per serving (1 bag)
Details: Yummy Hunters love this delicious chocolate-flavored tea, hot or cold. It makes loading up on liquids easy. *Helen:* I agree, keep pumping the fluids. *Eric:* Subtle but delicious.
Availability: Heath food stores and online

* Green Tea with Lemon
R.C. Bigelow, Green Tea with Lemon
R.C. Bigelow, Inc.
888 244-3569 www.bigelowtea.com
Bottom Line: 0 calories per serving (1 bag)
Details: Yummy Hunters talk about the wonderful flavor and how it rejuvenates them. *Helen:* Science and health writers praise the virtues of green tea. *Eric:* Strong and flavorful.
Availability: Supermarkets

* Panda Berry Tea
The Republic of Tea, Panda Berry Tea
The Republic of Tea
800-298-4832 www.republicoftea.com
Bottom Line: 5 calories per serving (1 bag)
Details: Yummy Hunters bought it for their children so they could drink tea like grown-ups. They now confess it's one of their favorites. They like that a percentage of the proceeds go to a school for abused and neglected children. *Helen & Eric:* Strong berry flavor with a hint of honey sweetness.
Availability: Supermarkets, health food stores, Borders, Barnes & Noble and online

* Sencha Green & White Tea
Long Life Organic Sencha Green & White Tea
Long Life Beverage Company
800-848-7331 www.long-life.com
Bottom Line: 0 calories per serving (1 bag)
Details: Yummy Hunters say it's a gem of a tea. *Helen & Eric:* Delicate and delicious.
Availability: Health food stores

We spend the first half of our lives wasting our health to gain wealth and the second half of our lives spending our wealth to gain our health.

BREAD

Bagels, Breads, Breadsticks, Croutons,
English Muffins, Taco Shells

Breads may be out of favor in some quarters,
but a sandwich just isn't a sandwich without
the bread. Our Yummy Hunters agree, and
fortunately they have discovered a variety of
superb choices that fit into most diet plans and
keep *sandwich* in the dictionary.

BAGELS

✱ Sesame Seed
Control-Carb Sesame Seed Bagel
Controlled Carb Gourmet Bakery
800-598-7720 www.controlledcarbgourmet.com
Bottom Line: 40 calories per serving (½ bagel)
Details: One Yummy Hunter took a chance on
these when she saw the low calorie count. It was
the best thing she could have done. *Helen:* I
toasted them and added lite cream cheese. It was
delish. *Eric:* I love a woman who's willing to take a
risk. Let's take our Yummy Hunter to Vegas!
Availability: Online at www.gethealthyamerica.com

✱ Sweet Wheat
Western, Alternative Bagel, Sweet Wheat
Western Bagel Baking Corp.
818-786-5847 www.westernbagel.com
Bottom Line: 110 calories per serving (1 bagel)
Details: One Yummy Hunter told us a friend served
these bagels at brunch and everyone was surprised
to learn they were low calorie. Others add the
unique, sweet wheat flavor makes them so tasty.
Helen & Eric: We also love the sweet wheat flavor
and think they taste like a fresh deli or bagel-store
bagel.
Availability: Online

* Whole Wheat
Western, Perfect 10
Western Bagel Baking Corp.
818-786-5847 www.westernbagel.com
Bottom Line: 140 calories per serving (2.5 oz)
Details: *Helen:* This is another of my discoveries.
Although they are higher in calories than other
bagels, they are more filling. We cut them in half
and melted two slices of Horizon Organic American
cheese on top with a little tomato sauce to make
delicious pizza bagels. As far as I'm concerned,
they are a perfect 10! *Eric:* Did Bo Derek makes
these? *Helen:* No, I did.
Availability: Online

BREADS

* Blueberry
Jacobsen's Snack Toast, Blueberry
Log House Foods
763-546-8395 www.loghousefoods.com
Bottom Line: 45 calories per serving (1 slice)
Details: Yummy Hunters eat them plain for
breakfast and say they're sweet, crunchy and truly
filling. *Helen:* A unique and wonderful-tasting
product. Stands on its own as a sweet treat. *Eric:* I
eat 'em right out of the box. We also tried the
Raspberry and Cinnamon Raisin, and they were
equally awesome.
Availability: Supermarkets and by phone

* Multigrain
Vermont Bread, Multigrain, Organic Bread
Vermont Bread & Baldwin Hill
800-721-4057
Bottom Line: 70 calories per serving (1 slice)
Details: Yummy Hunters say it goes great with jams
or cheese sandwiches. One Yummy Hunter just
started a diet and said she has a long way to go,
but this bread is making the journey easier. *Helen:*
Made our sandwiches of chicken breasts and
lettuce delectable. *Eric:* The nutty grains in this
bread make me nuts. *Helen:* So that explains it!

Availability: Health food stores on the East Coast, by phone and online at www.netgrocer.com

✳ Original
Flat Out Bread, Original
Flat Out Bread
866-944-5445 www.flatoutbread.com
Bottom Line: 210 calories per serving (1 piece)
Details: *Helen:* Thank you, Flat Out, for sending us these great-tasting wraps. *Eric:* Flat out delicious, especially wrapped around tuna salad.
Availability: Wal-Mart and Kroger supermarkets

✳ Raisin and Cinnamon
Mochi, Raisin and Cinnamon
Grainaissance
800-472-4697 www.grainaissance.com
Bottom Line: 120 calories per serving (1.5 oz)
Details: Yummy Hunters told us these are their favorite dinner rolls. One said her daughter loves to watch through the glass oven door as the rolls take shape. *Helen & Eric:* When we were told about this product, we were surprised at the solid, brick-like shape. However unappetizing the packaging may be, don't let its looks fool you. The rolls are delicious!
Availability: Selected supermarkets and health food stores

✳ Rye with Caraway Seeds
Arnold, Real Jewish Rye, Melba Thin
Arnold Foods Company, Inc.
973-785-7601 www.gwbakeries.com
Bottom Line: 110 calories per serving (2 slices)
Details: One Yummy Hunter brags she lost 80 pounds without giving up her Arnold's Real Jewish Rye bread. Another says he likes the caraway seeds and thinks thin is in, so this thinly sliced bread is his first choice. *Helen & Eric:* We toasted it up, smeared on some Better'n Peanut Butter and it made for a delicious sandwich.
Availability: Supermarkets and ordering online at www.netgrocer.com and www.shopfoodex.com

* Sesame
Suzie's Diet Tortilla Corn Flatbreads, Sesame
Wedgie Diabetic Foods
718-768-0821
Bottom Line: 95 calories per serving (3 flatbreads)
Details: *Helen:* I just discovered these flatbreads and now they are an indispensable part of my diet plan. I eat it with tuna salad, salmon and also cottage cheese on top. *Eric:* I ate them plain and they were very good. Then Helen tells me I should put something on them—but it was too late. I was full.
Availability: Online at www.gethealthyamerica.com

* 7 Grain
Pepperidge Farm, Light 7 Grain
Pepperidge Farm, Inc.
888-737-7374 www.campbellsoups.com
Bottom Line: 140 calories per serving (3 slices)
Details: Yummy Hunters love the wheaty, nutty flavor and eat it plain for breakfast and with turkey baloney for lunch. One declares she eats it all the time and still has lost weight and doesn't know why there is such an anti bread fuss going on. *Helen:* Exceptionally great-tasting textured sandwich bread. *Eric:* An abundance of rich flavor; great with all our favorite spreads.
Availability: Supermarket and ordering online at www.shopfoodex.com

* Wheat, Sprouted
Vermont Bread, Sprouted Wheat, All Natural Bread
Vermont Bread & Baldwin Hill
800-721-4057
Bottom Line: 60 calories per serving (1 slice)
Details: Yummy Hunters love to eat it plain or toasted. They even break it up and put it into their soft-boiled eggs. *Helen:* We agree with our Yummy Hunters, but we also used it to make French toast. *Eric:* I added a little Ginger People's Ginger Syrup. What a sweet treat!
Availability: Health food stores on the East Coast, by phone and online at www.netgrocer.com

✳ Whole Wheat
Damascus Bakeries, Roll-Up, Whole Wheat
Damascus Bakeries, Inc.
718-855-1456 www.damascusbakery.com
Bottom Line: 110 calories per serving (1 wrap)
Details: Yummy Hunters on low-carb diets say this is their bread salvation. One told us her kids call her "the Wrap Happy Mom." *Helen:* That nickname still has us laughing! Smaller than your normal-size wraps, but bigger on taste. *Eric:* This wrap knows how to wrap up the flavor.
Availability: Online and ordering at www.supplimentsstore.com

✳ Whole Wheat
Thomas', Sahara, Pita Bread, Whole Wheat
A Unit of George Weston Bakeries, Inc.
800-356-3314 www.gwbakeries.com
Bottom Line: 70 calories per serving (1 mini size pocket)
Details: Yummy Hunters say it makes sandwiches really delicious and they use it to hold tuna salads. *Helen:* We love to put veggies and cheese in it and mic the whole thing. *Eric:* The whole wheat flavor really makes this pita bread an outstanding choice.
Availability: Supermarkets and ordering online at www.netgrocer.com

✳ Whole Wheat, Honey
The Baker, Whole Wheat, Honey Rolls
The Baker
908-995-4040 www.the-baker.com
Bottom Line: 90 calories per serving (1 roll)
Details: Yummy Hunters say it has a wonderful honey flavor and complements the taste of their veggie burgers. They rave it's a family favorite. *Helen:* A full-size bun with a sweet flavor. The start to any great sandwich. *Eric:* We made tuna melts and brought new meaning to the term "hot cross buns."
Availability: Supermarkets, health food stores on the East Coast and online

* Whole Wheat, Potato
Martin's Famous, Whole Wheat, Potato Bread
Martin's Famous Pastry Shoppe, Inc.
800-548-1200 www.potatoroll.com
Bottom Line: 70 calories per serving (1 slice)
Details: Yummy Hunters say this is the best-tasting bread they have ever eaten and words alone cannot describe this delicious product.
Helen: I've never tasted anything quite like this. It's a whole wheat bread with a totally new twist.
Eric: How do you spell perfection? M-A-R-T-I-N-S
Availability: Online at www.netgrocer.com

* Whole Wheat, Potato
Martin's, Whole Wheat Potato Rolls
Martin's Famous Pastry Shoppe, Inc.
800-548-1200 www.potatoroll.com
Bottom Line: 80 calories per serving (1 roll)
Details: Yummy Hunters say this is more like a sweet roll. It makes either a great sandwich roll or you can munch on them right out of the bag.
Helen: This scrumptious bread has a lovely taste and you should try it ASAP. *Eric:* I put some Brummel & Brown yogurt on it. What a sweet distraction!
Availability: Online at www.netgrocer.com

BREADSTICKS

* Plain
Ricciole, Plain Breadsticks
Ricciole
908-862-5000
Bottom Line: 60 calories per serving (12 pieces)
Details: Yummy Hunters rave about the sweet taste but also love the weight and thickness of each stick. Others love the crunch and lightness of these breadsticks. *Helen:* How right they are. Goes great with any low-calorie salad dressing, spread or dip. *Eric:* I can't stop eating them. Somebody help me, please.
Availability: Supermarkets and by phone

* Sesame
Stella D'Oro, Breadsticks, Sesame
Kraft Foods, Inc.
888-878-3552 www.kraftfoods.com/stelladoro/
Bottom Line: 50 calories per serving (1 breadstick)
Details: Yummy Hunters like to dunk them into tuna and lite mayo mix. Another says a salad isn't a salad unless they can munch on one of these on the side. *Helen:* Light, crispy and the sesame seeds add plenty of oomph. *Eric:* Man, does this taste good with a smear of Brummel & Brown yogurt spread.
Availability: Some supermarkets; phone for store locations and online at www.netgrocer.com

* Traditional
Delallo, Traditional, Thin, Breadsticks
George E. Delallo Co. Inc.
800-433-9100 www.delallo.com
Bottom Line: 110 calories per serving (9 breadsticks)
Details: Yummy Hunters say they love to dunk them in salsa or spread on some low-cal cheese for a real snack treat. *Helen:* We dipped them in the Brummel & Brown Yogurt spread. What a delicious treat! *Eric:* Be warned. Once you start eating these, it's hard to stop!
Availability: Supermarkets and online

CROUTONS

* Garlic & Onion
Chatham Village, Garlic & Onion, Fat Free, Croutons
T. Marzetti Co.
614-846-2232 www.marzetti.com
Bottom Line: 30 calories per serving (2 tbsp)
Details: Yummy Hunters love the garlic and onion taste. They say it livens up any salad. *Helen:* The full garlic and onion flavor enhances the tastes of salads and soups. *Eric:* Just remember to brush your teeth afterward unless you're going to meet Dracula.
Availability: Supermarkets and online

ENGLISH MUFFINS

* English Muffins
Weight Watchers, English Muffins
A Unit of George Weston Bakeries, Inc.
800-356-3314 www.weightwatchers.com
Bottom Line: 100 calories per serving (1 muffin)
Details: Yummy Hunters on Weight Watchers love this 1-point wonder. *Helen:* I toasted it and let the Brummel & Brown melt its way through and it was delish. *Eric:* I second the motion.
Availability: Supermarkets and online at www.netgrocer.com

* Original
Thomas', Original, English Muffins
A Unit of George Weston Bakeries, Inc.
800-356-3314 www.gwbakeries.com
Bottom Line: 120 calories per serving (1 muffin)
Details: Yummy Hunters love the fact they can eat the entire muffin and not ruin their diets. One told us how important eating the whole muffin was because when she's eating with her family and only eats a portion of what's served, she feels singled out and penalized for being on a diet. *Helen:* Now one of my all-time childhood favorites is back on my breakfast menu. *Eric:* This is our favorite English muffin. Those flavor-catching nooks and crannies were made for soaking (butter and jelly, low-cal, of course).
Availability: Supermarkets and ordering online at www.netgrocer.com

(For all other muffins, go to the Muffins category.)

TACO SHELLS

* Taco
La Tiara, Taco Shells
Gladstone Food Products Co., Inc.
Gladstone MO 64118
Bottom Line: 31 calories per serving (1 shell)

Details: *Helen:* Eric grabbed a box on the recommendation of the store owner and we weren't disappointed. A thin crust that is light but jam-packed with flavor. We filled one up with lite shredded cheese, sliced tomatoes, sweet onions, salsa and we were good to go. *Eric:* Be warned, they are very thin, so shove them gently into your mouth or they will crumble in your hand and you will have to lick them up like a hungry dog. Woof, woof!
Availability: Online at www.gethealthyamerica.com and www.lowcarbnexus.com

Taco
Old El Paso, Taco Shells
General Mills, Inc.
800-999-7427 www.oldelpaso.com
Bottom Line: 150 calories per serving (3 shells)
Details: One Yummy Hunter says she takes ground turkey, adds her own secret taco recipe, and then stuffs it all into El Paso taco shells with some lite cheese and shredded lettuce. Another likes to crunch her lunch by putting smoked turkey, mustard and lite cheese in her shell. *Helen & Eric:* Our Yummy Hunter failed to share her taco recipe, so we made tuna tacos and the taco crunch really added some pick-me-up to the tuna.
Availability: Supermarkets

When I'm counting calories, crumbs don't count.

BREAKFAST MEATS

Iᴛ ᴜѕᴇᴅ ᴛᴏ ʙᴇ unless you were on a low-carb, high-protein diet this category of breakfast foods was sacrificed first. Thank goodness times have changed, as you can see by these Yummy, low-cal discoveries.

* Applewood Smoked Bacon

Wellshire Farms, Center Cut Bacon, Apple Smoked
Wellshire Farms
888-786-2331 www.wellshirefarms.com
Bottom Line: 60 calories per serving (2 slices)
Details: Yummy Hunters make this for the entire family and say it's everyone's favorite. They add, great with eggs, waffles or as a BLT. They love that it's all natural. *Eric:* Don't cook this up unless you want your neighbors beating down your door. Of course, you could tell them it doesn't taste half as good as it smells. Right.
Availability: Supermarkets and online

* Bacon

Betty Crocker, Bac-Os
General Mills, Inc.
800-828-3291 www.bettycrocker.com
Bottom Line: 30 calories per serving (1½ tbsp)
Details: Yummy Hunters put them in salads and eat them out of the jar. They happily inform us besides being low-cal and tasting just like bacon, they're also kosher. *Helen:* We made ourselves a Bac-Os omelette. *Eric:* Even if you don't like bacon, Bac-Os add an interesting, smoky flavor that's worth a taste. Oh boy, oh Bac-Os!
Availability: Supermarkets

✳ Bacon
Smart Bacon
Lightlife Foods
800-769-3279 www.lightlife.com
Bottom Line: 45 calories per serving (2 strips)
Details: Puts bacon back in their lives, rave overjoyed Yummy Hunters. They make Smart Bacon and egg-white omelettes and this rewarding meal motivates them to stay on their diets. *Helen:* They certainly do liven up eggs. We slapped the combo between slices of lite white and it made a great sandwich. *Eric:* We also made BLTs and couldn't agree more with our Yummy Hunters' glowing review.
Availability: Supermarkets, health food stores; store locations online

✳ Sausage
Healthy Choice, Breakfast Sausage
ConAgra Foods, Inc.
800-457-6649 www.healthychoice.com
Bottom Line: 70 calories per serving (3 patties)
Details: Yummy Hunters tell us they add them to eggs to make weekend brunches more like eating out. *Helen:* I let Eric wolf these down and he swears they let him pig out intelligently. *Eric:* Oink, oink!
Availability: Supermarkets

✳ Sausage Patties
Morningstar Farms, Veggie, Breakfast Sausage Patties
Kellogg Co.
800-557-6525 www.morningstarfarms.com
Bottom Line: 80 calories per serving (1 patty)
Details: Yummy Hunters say they like to throw them between two pieces of lite bread with a little mustard. They add it makes a great breakfast or lunch. *Helen:* We made a sausage LT and discovered it's the perfect combo to put on a breakfast bun. *Eric:* Looks like sausage, tastes like sausage. Whadayamean it's not sausage? *Helen:* Of course, it's sausage. It's a veggie sausage.
Availability: Supermarkets

✳ Turkey Bacon
Applegate Farms, Uncured, Turkey Bacon
Applegate Farms
866-587-5858 www.applegatefarms.com

Bottom Line: 38 calories per serving (1 slice)

Details: Yummy Hunters swear it tastes better than bacon and comes without the guilt. *Helen:* Its wonderfully smoky aroma makes cooking it a joy. It's sure to enhance any meal. *Eric:* True, smokehouse-turkey flavor that goes great with eggs or on a TBLT (Turkey, Bacon, Lettuce, & Tomato).

Availability: Health food stores; store locations and ordering online

I seem to gain weight from BLTs: bites, licks and tastes!

BURGERS & VEGGIE BURGERS

W HERE'S THE BEEF? Well, it's in the turkey, the soy and the chicken! Hooray!

Beef
White Castle, Microwaveable Hamburgers
White Castle Distributing, Inc.
800-843-2728 www.whitecastle.com
Bottom Line: 270 calories per serving (2 sandwiches)
Details: Yummy Hunters love the memories these hamburgers bring back, not to mention how much fun they are to eat. *Eric:* My high school pals and I had to drive from Manhattan up to the Bronx to get our hands on these beauties and now all I have to do is go to the microwave. Ain't progress swell!
Availability: Supermarkets

Chicken
Boca, Chik'n Patties
Boca Foods Company
www.bocaburger.com
Bottom Line: 160 calories per serving (1 patty)
Details: Yummy Hunters pick this because they like the spicy taste and it makes a great lunch or dinner for the entire family. *Helen & Eric:* We put them on a roll with a dab of lite mayo on one side and mustard on the other and had one heck of a burger.
Availability: Supermarkets, health and gourmet food stores; store locations online

Chicken
Morningstar Farms, Chik Patties
Kellogg Co.
800-557-6525 www.morningstarfarms.com
Bottom Line: 150 calories per serving (1 patty)
Details: Yummy Hunters say these patties have an authentic chicken taste. They put them on a lite bun with a little lettuce, tomato and ketchup and they're set for the afternoon. *Helen:* I served it to my family with a plate of pasta and it made for a tasty, satisfying meal. *Eric:* I like it either on lite bread or a bun. Any way you serve them, the taste is strong and flavorful.
Availability: Supermarkets

Fajita
Morningstar Farms, Fajita Burgers
Kellogg Co.
800-557-6525 www.morningstarfarms.com
Bottom Line: 130 calories per serving (1 burger)
Details: Yummy Hunters love this delicious variation that has a nice Mexican kick to it. One adds she likes putting it on a lite bun with lettuce and tomato. *Helen:* Mexican spice turns this veggie burger into something new and exciting. A real fiesta! *Eric:* Wonderfully exotic tasting and another reason to eat a veggie burger, not that I need one.
Availability: Supermarkets

✱ Garlic
Boca, Burgers, Roasted Garlic
Boca Foods Company
www.bocaburger.com
Bottom Line: 80 calories per serving (1 burger)
Details: Yummy Hunters warn these can be lethal, especially to kids who have been known to polish off a box before you can say Boca. *Helen:* Delightful garlicky taste adds a new and exciting twist to an already superior product. *Eric:* Like the man said, I never met a Boca Burger I didn't like.
Availability: Supermarkets, health and gourmet food stores; store locations online

* Grilled Vegetable
Boca, Burgers, Grilled Vegetable
Boca Foods Company
www.bocaburger.com
Bottom Line: 70 calories per serving (1 burger)
Details: Yummy Hunters love the outstanding flavor and how these burgers always satisfy their appetites. Some eat them plain with tomatoes on the side; others like them the more traditional way on a lite bun with ketchup. *Helen:* Fire up the grill for this delicious veggie sensation. *Eric:* Another Boca bonanza!
Availability: Supermarkets, health and gourmet food stores; store locations online

* Harvest
Morningstar Farms, Veggie, Harvest Burgers
Kellogg Co.
800-557-6525 www.morningstarfarms.com
Bottom Line: 140 calories per serving (1 burger)
Details: Yummy Hunters say this very filling burger has it all. Another adds it has taste, texture and always satisfies. *Helen:* The garden-fresh veggie taste makes this one superior burger. Try two of these with a slice of low-fat American cheese in the center for a bunless burger sensation. *Eric:* Don't need any condiments on this baby.
Availability: Supermarkets

* Plain
Boca, Ground Meatless Burger, Plain
Boca Foods Company
www.bocaburger.com
Bottom Line: 60 calories per serving (½ cup)
Details: One Yummy Hunter told us how he opens a can of stewed tomatoes, adds fresh garlic, pours it over the ground burger with spaghetti squash on the side and he's in heaven. *Helen:* We added a little ketchup, garlic salt and made sloppy joes. *Eric:* Once again, we bow to Boca!
Availability: Supermarkets, health and gourmet food stores; store locations online

✳ Spicy Black Bean
Morningstar Farms, Veggie Burgers, Spicy Black Bean
Kellogg Co.
800-557-6525 www.morningstarfarms.com
Bottom Line: 150 calories per serving (1 burger)
Details: A Yummy Hunter of Spanish descent loves to make these for her family because they remind her of her mother's delicious bean dish. Another says this burger enabled her to lose those extra 10 pounds. *Helen & Eric:* Spicy, south-of-the-border flavor makes this a wickedly special treat.
Availability: Supermarkets

Tomato & Basil
Morningstar Farms, Veggie, Pizza Burgers, Tomato & Basil
Kellogg Co.
800-557-6525 www.morningstarfarms.com
Bottom Line: 130 calories per serving (1 burger)
Details: Yummy Hunters say this is another food that has helped them to stay on their diets. They add it has a superb pizza taste and it's the perfect choice when they want something quick and easy. *Helen:* We gobbled them up like kids, washing them down with a nice tall glass of Mistic Wild Cherry. *Eric:* This Yummy burger has just the right amount of seasoning to make you drool with delight.
Availability: Supermarkets

Turkey
Perdue, Turkey Burgers
Perdue
800-473-7383 www.perdue.com
Bottom Line: 160 calories per serving cooked (1 burger)
Details: Yummy Hunters like the convenience. The premade patties go straight from freezer to grill and always taste great and make a meal the entire family enjoys. *Helen:* Nice to have a delicious, preseasoned, portion-controlled turkey burger. *Eric:* These Yummy burgers remove the guesswork at mealtime and make dieting easy.
Availability: Supermarkets

* Veggie Pizza
Dr. Praeger's, Veggie Pizza Burgers
Ungar's Food Products
201-703-1300 www.drpraegers.com
Bottom Line: 120 calories per serving (1 burger)
Details: Yummy Hunters claim this is the ultimate pizza burger. *Helen:* This is what you get when you cross the perfect veggie burger with the ultimate pizza seasoning. *Eric:* This is one doctor that knows how to doctor-up a great veggie burger.
Availability: Some supermarkets; store locations online

* Veggie Royale
Dr. Praeger's, California Burgers, Veggie Royale
Ungar's Food Products
201-703-1300 www.drpraegers.com
Bottom Line: 100 calories per serving (1 burger)
Details: Yummy Hunters rave they're the best veggie burgers, ever. They add they're jam-packed with all sorts of fresh vegetables that make them special. *Helen & Eric:* Exploding with tasty veggies makes this one amazing burger.
Availability: Some supermarkets; store locations online and ordering at www.hillersmarket.com

Nothing tastes as good as thin feels.

CAKE

Oh, to be able to have our cake and eat it, too! Here are some Yummy low-calorie options that enable you to enjoy the birthday celebration, have something to serve at the weekly card game or just savor when you're having a cup of coffee.

---

* Angel Food
Hostess, Angel Food Cake
Interstate Brands Companies
816-502-4000 www.interstatebakeries.com
Bottom Line: 160 calories per serving (⅕ cake)
Details: Our Yummy Hunters say Hostess makes a fluffy and delicious angel food cake. They like to slice it, put on fresh strawberries, a little bit of Cool Whip and make their own strawberry shortcake. *Helen & Eric:* We were no angels when it came to portion control on this baby.
Availability: Online at www.hometown-treats.com

* Angel Food
Little Debbie, Angel Food, Raspberry Filled Cakes
McKee Foods
800-522-4499 www.littledebbie.com
Bottom Line: 110 calories per serving (1 cake)
Details: Our Yummy Hunters love this product to death. They say the raspberry filling makes this one special cake. *Helen & Eric:* We bit into this cake and the raspberry filling provided such a sweet sensation that both Eric and I simply nodded our heads and smiled from ear to ear.
Availability: Supermarkets

* Apple Spice
Harry and David, Low-fat, Dessert Cakes, Apple Spice
Harry and David
877-322-1200 www.harryanddavid.com
Bottom Line: 210 calories per serving (¼ cake)
Details: One Yummy Hunter told us she selects one for her family and freezes the rest. Her favorite was the apple spice cake. *Helen & Eric:* We couldn't pick a favorite. Other flavors are Orange, Lemon-Raspberry and Chocolate-Cherry.
Availability: Harry and David locations and online

Cheese Cake, Chocolate or Strawberry
Chatila's Bakery Cheesecake
Chatila's Bakery
877-619-5398 www.chatilasbakery.com
Bottom Line: 40 calories per serving (1.6-oz cup)
Details: *Helen & Eric:* A Yummy Hunter wrote to us about Chatila's bakery muffins (which are in the muffins chapter). We contacted the bakery, learned about their famous cheesecakes and now we have two reasons to thank our Yummy Hunter.
Availability: Online

* Coffee Cakes
Drake's, Low Fat, Coffee Cakes
Interstate Brands Companies
800-483-7253 www.drakescake.com
Bottom Line: 110 calorie per serving (1 cake)
Details: Our Yummy Hunters tell us they love to slice the cakes into halves and then soak them in their coffee. *Helen:* Warning, do not open this double pack without a friend. *Eric:* Low in fat, sky high in taste.
Availability: Online at www.hometown-treats.com

Dieting is not a piece of cake.

CANDY

Candy is one food that has questionable nutritional value, but that never stopped us. Let's face it, candy satisfies our emotional needs, and when we're dieting, it's all about emotions. You will be delighted to know the following foods hold back the calories without reining in our emotions.

＊ Butter Cream Caramel
Weight Watchers Crispy Butter Cream Caramel
Whitman's
800-477-8683 www.whitmans.com
Bottom Line: 50 calories per serving (1 piece)
Details: Yummy Hunters love these gooey, portion-controlled candies that not only satisfy but are filling. *Helen:* Crispy, chewy and oh, soo chocolatey. *Eric:* These are unbelievably good. One of my favorite after-dinner treats.
Availability: Supermarkets and drug stores

＊ Chocolate, Dark
Chambers Farms, Tosted, Gourmet Sweet Dark Chocolate Clusters
Chambers Farms
888-526-9296 www.tosteds.com
Bottom Line: 48 calories per serving (1 cluster)
Details: Yummy Hunters delight in this deliciously rich, chocolate treat. *Helen:* The combo of nuts and dark chocolate creates an incredible gourmet treat. *Eric:* Without a doubt, my absolute favorite new chocolate candy of 2006.
Availability: Online

Chocolate Almond
Splurge!, Chocolate Almond Bar
Proto Health Innovations
877-677-6677 www.protohealthealth.com
Bottom Line: 140 calories per serving (1 oz)
Details: Yummy Hunters say they can now pass up the candy counter at movies when they arm themselves with this deliciously satisfying sweet treat. *Helen:* True to its name this is one candy worth the splurge. *Eric:* Finely chopped almonds combined with delicious chocolate make this an irresistible choice.
Availability: Online

* Chocolate & Caramel Creme
Kraft Foods, Sugar Free Creme Savers Hard Candy, Chocolate & Caramel Creme
Kraft Foods, Inc.
800-244-4596 www.candystand.com
Bottom Line: 45 calories per serving (5 pieces)
Details: Yummy Hunters love the caramel, creamy flavor. Others declare they always need something sweet after a meal and one or two of these do the trick. *Helen:* Great after-meal sweet and they don't taste diet at all. Also available in strawberries and creme, which are just as Yummy. *Eric:* I like to roll them around in my mouth. OK, so I'm a little strange.
Availability: Supermarkets and drugstores

* Chocolate Mint
Go Lightly, Sugar Free, Chocolate Mint Candy
Hillside Candy
800-524-1304 www.hillsidecandy.com
Bottom Line: 45 calories per serving (4 pieces)
Details: Yummy Hunters love the chocolate, minty combo and say they always put these candies out for company. *Helen:* The combination of mint and chocolate is a refreshing sensation. The flavor lasts long after the candy is gone. *Eric:* Another one of those addicting products. So, go lightly.
Availability: Supermarkets, drugstores, Wal-Mart and online at www.jambsupply.com

Cookie Dough, Peanut Butter
Carb Slim, Cookie Dough, Peanut Butter Spice
Breakthrough Engineered Nutrition
800-689-2831 www.carbslim.com
Bottom Line: 105 calories per serving (28 g)
Details: Yummy Hunters say when dieting, they crave something sweet after meals but find it hard to find something small in calories and big in taste. This fits the bill. *Helen:* This terrific peanut butter treat put a smile on this cookie dough lover! *Eric:* What a great combo. My money's on this cookie dough.
Availability: Supermarkets, Wal-Mart, GNC, Vitamin Shoppe and online

✱ Fruit
SunRidge Farms, Organic Sunny Bears
SunRidge Farms
831-462-1280   www.sunridgefarms.com
Bottom Line: 130 calories per serving (17 pieces)
Details: Yummy Hunters say it gives them a fruit-filled taste sensation. *Helen:* Cute little bear - shaped candies with a light sugar coating bursts with sweet flavor in your mouth. I love the fact that you get 17 pieces to a serving. I ate them really slowly and my sweet tooth was in heaven for a really long time. Yum, Yum! *Eric:* The flavor of these bears will never go into hibernation. How sweet they are!
Availability: Supermarkets, health food stores and online

✱ Fruit Snacks
Planet Harmony, Fruit Snacks
Harmony Foods Corporation
800-837-2855 www.harmonyfoods.com
Bottom Line: 130 calories per serving (12 pieces)
Details: Yummy Hunters find it hard to stop once they eat one but tell us the delicious flavor is well worth it. *Helen:* Mouth-wateringly wonderful. *Eric:* Juicy, juicy, juicy. Did I forget to say they were juicy?
Availability: Health food stores

✳ Ginger
Ginger People, Original, Ginger Chews
Royal Pacific Foods
800-551-5284 www.gingerpeople.com
Bottom Line: 40 calories per serving (2 pieces)
Details: Yummy Hunters confess this is a most unusual but delicious sweet treat. Others who are ginger lovers gush over this chewy delight. *Helen:* A delicious and long-lasting sweet-tasting delicacy. *Eric:* I can't decide whether it's better to chew right into it and let the sweet ginger flavor make all my taste buds explode at once or just suck on it and let the juices wake up those buds, one at a time until I go into ginger arrest.
Availability: Online

✳ Gummy Bears
Planet Harmony, Gummy Bears
Harmony Foods Corporation
800-837-2855 www.harmonyfoods.com
Bottom Line: 120 calories per serving (17 pieces)
Details: Yummy Hunters tell us how terrific they are to take along in the car when you want to have a long-lasting sweet treat. *Helen:* I like these a lot. They are a real favorite of mine. *Eric:* Ever try to chew down on them so your top and bottom teeth stick together, all the while you drain the juice out of these babies?
Availability: Health food stores

✳ Jelly Beans
Harry and David Sugar Free Jelly Beans
Harry and David
800-547-3033 www.harryanddavid.com
Bottom Line: 90 calories per serving (2 tbsp)
Details: Yummy Hunters say this is the perfect munchy at work. They eat them one at a time and if they eat them slow enough, they can get through an entire afternoon. *Helen:* Each flavor is a taste sensation! *Eric:* After days and nights of endless experimentation I discovered the perfect two-flavor combo. I am now busily at work at seeing which three flavors go best with each other.

Availability: Harry and David locations and online

* Licorice
Panda, Fat Free, Licorice
New World Marketing Group
203-221-8008 www.panda.fi
Bottom Line: 110 calories per serving (1 bar)
Details: Yummy Hunters who loved licorice as a kid, go wild for this great-tasting licorice. *Helen & Eric:* Flavor really lasts and keeps you from reaching for more food.
Availability: Health food stores and online at www.candyfavorites.com, www.shopnatural.com, www.truefoodsmarket.com

* Marshmallow
La Nouba, Marshmallows
La Nouba, Inc.
866-967-8477 www.lanouba.be
Bottom Line: 15.3 calories per serving (7.5 g)
Details: When Yummy Hunters are dying for something sweet and delicious, they pop one or two of these in their mouths. They add, these marshmallows are nice and fluffy. *Helen:* Tastes like real marshmallows to us. *Eric:* Sweet and delicious, but like the other La Nouba products, heed the label and watch excessive consumption — it could cause a laxative effect on your system.
Availability: Health food stores and some supermarkets

Mint Dark Chocolate
Gayle's Miracles, the Perfect Chocolate Truffle, Mint Dark Chocolate
Gorant Candies, Inc.
800-572-4139 www.gaylesmiracles.com
Bottom Line: 30 calories per serving (1 piece)
Details: Yummy Hunters rave and rave about how wonderfully delicious these candies taste. *Helen:* Light and creamy and the perfect complement to any meal. *Eric:* These truffles are not to be trifled with! My God, they are good!
Availability: Online and at www.yummydelights.com

Peanut Butter
Peter Pan Wafers, Peanut Butter
Simply Lite Foods Corp.
800-753-4282 www.sweetnlowcandy.com
Bottom Line: 150 calories per serving (3 bars)
Details: Yummy Hunters love the great
combination of chocolate and peanut butter in a
wafer bar. *Helen:* A chocolate-covered light wafer
with a smooth, peanut butter flavor. A true
dessert. *Eric:* A doubly delicious combo. What's not
to love!
Availability: Supermarkets and drugstores

Peanut Butter Chocolate
Reese's, Sugar-Free, Peanut Butter Cups
Hershey Food Corp.
800-468-1714 www.reesespb.com
Bottom Line: 170 calories per serving (5 pieces)
Details: Yummy Hunters can't tell the difference
between the regular and sugar-free products. They
add they're watching their sugar intake, so they're
overjoyed they can continue to eat, in moderation,
of course, their favorite candy. *Helen:* What's to
say—we just love them. *Eric:* Really sweet and
delicious combination of chocolate and peanut
butter. As the bag states, you have to watch
excessive consumption because it can have a
laxative effect.
Availability: Supermarkets and drugstores

Peppermint
Newman's Own Organics, Peppermint Cups
Newman's Own Organics, The Second Generation
www.newmansownorganics.com
Bottom Line: 170 calories per serving (1 pckg)
Details: Yummy Hunters say this is their favorite
peppermint candy. Another simply says,
"Outstanding!" *Helen:* My mouth is watering just
thinking about how good these peppermint cups
taste. *Eric:* My cup runneth over with dark
chocolate and tasty peppermint.
Availability: Supermarkets and health food stores;
store locations and ordering online

✳ S'Mores, Marshmallow Creme
Hershey's, S'Mores, SnackBarz, Marshmallow Creme
Hershey Food Corp.
800-468-1714 www.hersheys.com/snackbarz
Bottom Line: 110 calories per serving (1 bar)
Details: Yummy Hunters rave about this delicious-tasting sandwich bar. *Helen:* It's a sandwich with creme in the middle, how good is that! *Eric:* You won't be able to resist the taste of the marshmallow creme.
Availability: Supermarkets and drugstores

✳ Strawberry
Fruities, Strawberry
Weight Watchers International
800-815-8704 www.weightwatchers.com
Bottom Line: 17 calories per serving (3 pieces)
Details: Yummy Hunters bought them at a Weight Watchers meeting and can't live without them. They buy half a dozen packs to keep on hand. *Helen:* We agree—they are delicious. Beware, Weight Watchers keeps changing the flavors, so stock up on your favorites and check our website for product replacements. *Eric:* I love to roll these fruities around on my tongue and then give them a big chew to get the juicy flavor in one quick spurt.
Availability: Weight Watchers Meeting Centers; center locations online

✳ Strawberry, Orange, Raspberry
Baskin-Robbins, Sugar-Free, Fruit Medley, Strawberry, Orange, Raspberry
Bestsweet, Inc.
888-211-5530 www.bestsweet.com
Bottom Line: 40 calories per serving (4 pieces)
Details: Yummy Hunters say they taste like their favorite Baskin-Robbins flavors. *Helen:* Fruity and delicious. Flavor that lasts a long time. *Eric:* How can they get the taste of ice cream in these tiny little candies? Any ideas, please write me.
Availability: Supermarkets, drugstores, Wal-Mart and ordering online at www.clorders.com

✱ Tootsie Roll
Tootsie Roll Pops
Tootsie Roll Industries, Inc.
www.tootsie.com
Bottom Line: 60 calories per serving (1 pop)
Details: Yummy Hunters say these pops bring back childhood memories. Only 1 point on Weight Watchers. One Yummy Hunter lost 25 pounds and eating these pops really helped. *Helen & Eric:* Bring a bag to the movies. They last longer than popcorn and, oh, how much sweeter.
Availability: Supermarkets

> *Inside some of us is a thin person struggling to get out, but that person can usually be sedated with a few pieces of chocolate.*

CEREAL – COLD

Nothing gives you quite the bang for the buck like cold cereals. You eat 'em in the morning with milk, snack on them in the afternoon right out of the box and use them as topping on your favorite low-fat yogurt.

———

Apple Cinnamon
Zoe, Flax and Granola Cereal, Apple Cinnamon
Zoe Foods
781-453-9000 www.zoefoods.com
Bottom Line: 190 calories per serving (½ cup)
Details: Yummy Hunters never experienced anything so deliciously satisfying. One adds that you can really get full on this wonderful cereal. *Helen:* The apple cinnamon makes it one of the most interesting granolas we've tasted. *Eric:* Delightful combo of flavors.
Availability: Supermarkets, health food stores, by phone at 800-233-3668 and online

✳ Banana Berry
Kellogg's, Fruit Harvest, Banana Berry
Kellogg Co.
800-962-1516 www.kelloggs.com
Bottom Line: 120 calories per serving (¾ cup)
Details: Yummy Hunters enjoy the sweetness of the dry bananas and berries; it's one of their favorites. *Helen:* Flakes are transformed by the harvest of fruit. *Eric:* Berry, berry good.
Availability: Supermarkets

✴ Banana Nut Multibran
Back to Nature, Banana Nut Multibran
Back to Nature
866-536-6946 www.backtonaturefoods.com
Bottom Line: 140 calories per serving (¾ cup)
Details: Yummy Hunters say there's a lot going on in this great-tasting cereal. They add it's got just the right combo of fruit and fiber. *Helen:* No doubt about it, my hat's off to our Yummy Hunters. *Eric:* Just tried it with 8th Continent's Vanilla Soy Milk and it was so good, I'm thinking next time I'll freeze it and serve it as a dessert!
Availability: Health food stores and Whole Foods

✴ Bran
General Mills, Fiber One, Bran Cereal
General Mills, Inc.
800-328-1140 www.generalmills.com
Bottom Line: 60 calories per serving (½ cup)
Details: Yummy Hunters who love bran say this cereal provides a subtle, sweet taste. They add fiber is a must when they diet. *Helen:* Good with milk, but it's also a delightful crunchy treat right out of the box. *Eric:* I'm one with Fiber One.
Availability: Supermarkets and ordering online at www.netgrocer.com

✴ Brown Rice Crisps
Barbara's, Brown Rice Crisps
Barbara's For A Brighter Future
707-765-2273 www.barbarasbakery.com
Bottom Line: 110 calories per serving (1 cup)
Details: Yummy Hunters love the light crunchiness of these crisps. *Helen:* Strong flavor but not overpowering, light yet filling. This cereal has definitely become one of our top five favorites. *Eric:* Great with sliced banana and peaches. Hats off to Barbara for another winner. Every year she gets more creative with her cereal ideas.
Availability: Health food stores and some supermarkets; store locations online and ordering at www.leesmarket.com

✳ Cinnamon
Barbara's, Puffins, Cinnamon
Barbara's For A Brighter Future
707-765-2273 www.barbarasbakery.com
Bottom Line: 100 calories per serving (¾ cup)
Details: *Helen:* A marvelously unique concept. I love the square, puffy shapes that float on top of the milk and never seem to sink. *Eric:* A fun cereal I enjoy with or without milk. Hats off to Helen for finding this wonderful cereal!
Availability: Health food stores and some supermarkets; store locations online and ordering at www.leesmarket.com and www.netgrocer.com

✳ Cinna-Raisin Crunch
Kashi, Good Friends, Cinna-Raisin Crunch
Kashi Company
858-274-8870 www.kashi.com
Bottom Line: 170 calories per serving (1 cup)
Details: Yummy Hunters love the taste, love the calorie count and love the fiber. *Helen:* Perfect combination of ingredients and flavors. *Eric:* A must-have if you love cinnamon and raisins, and who doesn't love cinnamon and raisins.
Availability: Supermarkets, health food stores, ordering online and at www.leesmarket.com

✳ Honey Clusters
General Mills, Fiber One, Bran Cereal
General Mills, Inc.
800-328-1140 www.generalmills.com
Bottom Line: 170 calories per serving (1¼ cup)
Details: One Yummy Hunter tells us her doctor is overjoyed that she is now eating this fiber-rich cereal. Others add not only is it filling, but they love the sweet taste and say it makes getting their fiber "fun." *Helen:* Great high-fiber cereal with just the right amount of sweetness. Half the serving amount was plenty for me. *Eric:* The box said I could have a whole serving and that's what I had. Still one with Fiber One.
Availability: Supermarkets and ordering online at www.netgrocer.com

✳ Multigrain
Health Valley, Organic Fiber, 7 Multigrain Flakes
Hain Celestial Group, Inc.
800-423-4846 www.hain-celestial.com
Bottom Line: 100 calories per serving (¾ cup)
Details: Yummy Hunters recommend adding a little lite syrup. Others prefer to sweeten their cereal with fruit. *Helen:* Great, tasty grains that stand on their own. *Eric:* It's not just flakes — it's texture, it's taste, it's terrific.
Availability: Supermarkets, health food stores and ordering online at www.leesmarket.com and www.naturemart.com

Oats & Honey
Cascadian Farm, Oats & Honey, Granola
General Mills, Inc.
800-624-4123 www.cascadianfarm.com
Bottom Line: 230 calories per serving (⅔ cup)
Details: Yummy Hunters say it's sweet as candy. One grabs a handful on the way out and eats it in the car. *Helen:* Granola doesn't always give you the biggest caloric bang for the buck, but this one is big on flavor, so it's worth the trade-off. *Eric:* It's one honey of a granola.
Availability: Supermarkets and health food stores; store locations online

Oat Bran
Kellogg's, Cracklin' Oat Bran
Kellogg Co.
800-962-1516 www.kelloggs.com
Bottom Line: 140 calories per serving (¾ cup)
Details: Yummy Hunters tell us it's high in fiber, has only 15 grams of sugar and still tastes like a supersweet dessert snack. One measures portions out in little bags so when she wants something sweet, she has a preportioned snack. *Helen:* To die for, but watch out for those calories. By the way, Eric has no self-control. *Eric:* I won't dignify Helen's remarks except to say, sometimes you have to give up control to get control.
Availability: Supermarkets

✳ A Low-Fat Product

✱ Raisins and Apples
Kashi, Medley, Raisins and Apples
Kashi Company
858-274-8870 www.kashi.com
Bottom Line: 120 calories per serving (¾ cup)
Details: Yummy Hunters eat it every day and tell us
it's one of the reasons they're losing weight. *Helen:*
The sweetness of the raisins and apples makes this
cereal a true delight. *Eric:* This medley makes
beautiful music.
Availability: Supermarkets, health food stores,
ordering online and at www.leesmarket.com and
www.netgrocer.com

✱ Rice
Health Valley, Rice Crunch-Ems!
Hain Celestial Group, Inc.
800-423-4846 www.hain-celestial.com
Bottom Line: 110 calories per serving (1 cup)
Details: Yummy Hunters tell us this cereal is
nothing short of perfection. *Helen:* The woven
texture of the square puffs allows the milk to flow
through and gives the cereal a really delicious,
milky rice flavor. *Eric:* I love it with sliced bananas
for breakfast. Really delicious.
Availability: Health food stores, some
supermarkets, online at www.leesmarket.com,
www.naturemart.com and www.netgrocer.com

✱ Seven Whole Grains & Sesame
Kashi, Go Lean, Seven Whole Grains & Sesame
Kashi Company
858-274-8870 www.kashi.com
Bottom Line: 140 calories per serving (¾ cup)
Details: A Yummy Hunter says she eats this every
morning with a sliced banana and has been losing
two pounds a week. *Helen:* Kudos to our
Yummy Hunter, and good luck. Another terrific
combination of grains that provides great taste.
Eric: Go lean, girl, go!
Availability: Supermarkets, health food stores,
ordering online and at www.leesmarket.com and
www.netgrocer.com

∗ Seven Whole Grains & Sesame
Kashi, Puffed Seven Whole Grains & Sesame
Kashi Company
858-274-8870 www.kashi.com
Bottom Line: 70 calories per serving (1 cup)
Details: Yummy Hunters who want volume say this is the best bang for the buck. *Helen:* I need to slice a half banana into mine to give it some sweetness. *Eric:* I sweeten it up with yogurt.
Availability: Supermarkets, health food stores, ordering online and at www.leesmarket.com and www.netgrocer.com

∗ Whole Grain
Life, Whole Grain Quaker Oats
The Quaker Oats Company
800-234-6281 www.lifecereal.com
Bottom Line: 120 calories per serving (½ cup)
Details: Yummy Hunters say these little squares are packed with sweetness. *Helen:* This old-time favorite of mine is so good, I eat it right out of the box. *Eric:* For the life of me, I don't know how they get it to taste so good.
Availability: Supermarkets, health food stores and online

∗ Whole Grain
Nature's Path, Heritage Bites, Whole Grain
Nature's Path
888-808-9505 www.naturespath.com
Bottom Line: 100 calories per serving (¾ cup)
Details: Yummy Hunters love this delicious cereal and say it saves them from slaving over a hot stove. *Helen:* The interesting woven texture allows the milk to seep right in. *Eric:* Provides the perfect amount of milk and Yummy cereal in every bite.
Availability: Supermarket and health food stores; store locations online and ordering at www.leesmarket.com

The only people who say fat people are jolly are skinny.

∗ A Low-Fat Product

CEREAL – HOT

NOTHING IS MORE DELICIOUS or more comforting on a cold winter's morning than oatmeal. The mixing of grains now makes that timeless classic more full-flavored and pleasing to the palate. For all those who have never had a taste for hot cereals, try these — you'll like them!

* Apples and Cinnamon
Quaker, Lower Sugar, Instant Oatmeal, Apples and Cinnamon
The Quaker Oats Company
800-555-6287 www.quakeroatmeal.com
Bottom Line: 110 calories per serving (1 packet)
Details: Yummy Hunters say easy-to-make warm, sweet breakfast makes their morning. *Helen & Eric:* All we have to say is — Apple Pie In A Bowl Of Oatmeal!
Availability: Supermarkets

* Banana Nut Barley
Fantastic, Oatmeal Big Cereal Cup, Banana Nut Barley
Fantastic Foods, Inc.
800-288-1089 www.fantasticfoods.com
Bottom Line: 270 calories per serving (70-g container)
Details: Yummy Hunters rave about this cereal's fabulous, nutty flavor. They add that it's very filling with a perfect texture, a great on-the-go food. *Helen & Eric:* Truly, the easiest, tastiest way to eat a healthy breakfast!
Availability: Supermarkets, health food stores and club stores; store locations and ordering online

✱ Cinnamon Roll
McCann's, Instant Irish Oatmeal, Cinnamon Roll
US Agent Paul Germann & Associates, Inc.
pga@webspan.net www.mccanns.ie
Bottom Line: 100 calories per serving (1 packet)
Details: *Helen & Eric:* We can't thank McCann's enough for the three, new, sugar-free instant oatmeals now on the market. Whether it's Maple and Brown Sugar, Apple and Cinnamon or the Cinnamon Roll, they all add up to delicious.
Availability: Supermarkets and online at www.netgrocer.com and www.efoodpantry.com

✱ Cream of Wheat
Nabisco, Instant Cream of Wheat
Nabisco, Inc.
800-622-4726 www.creamofwheat.com
Bottom Line: 90 calories per serving (1 pouch)
Details: Yummy Hunters bring this to work and say it's a convenient and satisfying breakfast and stops them from going out to the donut truck. *Helen:* This box has premeasured pouches, but the product also comes in containers, so check those boxes for serving size information. *Eric:* If you're a cream of wheat lover, you'll love the convenience of these easy-to-carry packages.
Availability: Supermarkets and ordering online at www.netgrocer.com

✱ Maple & Brown Sugar
Quaker, Lower Sugar, Instant Oatmeal, Maple & Brown Sugar
The Quaker Oats Company
800-555-6287 www.quakeroatmeal.com
Bottom Line: 120 calories per serving (1 packet)
Details: One oatmeal-loving Yummy Hunter says eating oatmeal for breakfast has helped her to lose 20 pounds. She adds that oatmeal in the morning fills her up. The sweetness makes this breakfast so enjoyable. *Helen:* What a sweet success story. Keep up the good work. *Eric:* Great way to start the day.
Availability: Supermarkets

* Maple Raisin, Grain
Fantastic, Maple Raisin 3-Grain Oatmeal, Big Cereal Cup, Maple Raisin, Grain
Fantastic Foods, Inc.
800-288-1089 www.fantasticfoods.com
Bottom Line: 270 calories per serving (78-g container)
Details: Yummy Hunters love the plump and moist raisins that give this cereal its mouth-watering flavor. They add they like that it's low in fat. *Helen & Eric:* Sweet and delicious, the combo of flavors and grains makes this a must-have breakfast.
Availability: Supermarkets, health food stores and club stores; store locations and ordering online

* Oat Bran
Hodgson, Oat Bran, Hot Cereal
Hodgson Mill, Inc.
800-525-0177 www.hodgsonmill.com
Bottom Line: 120 calories per serving (¼ cup dry)
Details: Yummy Hunters who love bran find warmth in this delicious and filling breakfast. *Helen:* We had a bowl with raisins and it was like eating a bran muffin right out of the oven. *Eric:* Sue me, I added chocolate soy milk to this too and made a chocolate bran muffin. *Helen:* Our next book is going to be called "Eric's Guide to the Many Uses of Chocolate Soy Milk."
Availability: Some supermarkets, by phone, online and at www.netgrocer.com

* Oatmeal
McCann's, Steel Cut, Irish Oatmeal
US Agent Paul Germann & Associates, Inc.
pga@webspan.net www.mccanns.ie
Bottom Line: 150 calories per serving (¼ cup dry)
Details: Yummy Hunters rave this cereal is the end all, be all. *Helen:* Extremely flavorful cereal because of the unique type of oats and the way it is cut. *Eric:* Oatmeal lovers will dance a jig after eating this Irish delight.
Availability: Supermarkets and online at www.efoodpantry.com, www.leesmarket.com and www.netgrocer.com

✱ Rice
Arrowhead Mills, Rice & Shine
Hain Celestial Group, Inc.
800-749-0730 www.arrowheadmills.com
Bottom Line: 150 calories per serving (¼ cup)
Details: Yummy Hunters love rice any way they can get it, so this is a nice alternative to oatmeal. *Helen:* Very creamy and tasty. *Eric:* Love the product name almost as much as I love the taste.
Availability: Supermarkets, some health food stores and ordering online at www.netgrocer.com

✱ 7 Grain Cereal
Fiddlers Green Farm, Island Choice, 7 Grain Cereal
Fiddlers Green Farm
800-729-7935 www.fiddlersgreenfarm.com
Bottom Line: 180 calories per serving (1 cup prepared)
Details: One Yummy Hunter said this cereal helps to fill her up in the morning, an important consideration during her first days of dieting. *Helen & Eric:* No matter how long you cook it, it always has a great grainy crunch and makes for a consistently delicious hot cereal.
Availability: Health food stores, by phone and online

Oh, this is just fun fat (I have a lot of fun).

CHEESE

Now you have a reason to smile and say cheese because our Yummy Hunters have discovered cheese that really tastes like cheese.

———

* American Cheese
Horizon, Organic American Singles
WhiteWave Food Companies
888-494-3020 www.horizonorganics.com
Bottom Line: 60 calories per serving (1 slice)
Details: Yummy Hunters say this is the cheese to use when they treat themselves to their all-time favorite grilled cheese and tomato sandwiches. *Helen & Eric:* We did the same, except we added turkey bacon and a little mustard.
Availability: Supermarkets and health food stores

* Babybel
The Laughing Cow, Mini Babybel, Light
Bel/Kaukauna USA, Inc.
920-788-3524 www.thelaughingcow.com
Bottom Line: 50 calories per serving (1 piece)
Details: Our Yummy Hunters say this fun little cheese takes the edge off their appetite. *Helen:* When dieting, this is so important because the last thing you want to do is sit down to a meal super hungry. *Eric:* Since I was a kid I thought Laughing Cow was the best name ever thought up for a product. Oh, right—great cheese flavor.
Availability: Supermarkets and ordering online at www.netgrocer.com

* Cheddar
Galaxy Nutritional Foods, Veggy Singles, Cheddar
Galaxy Nutritional Foods
407-855-5500 www.veggieforlife.com
Bottom Line: 60 calories per serving (1½ slices)
Details: Yummy Hunters who are vegetarian say they live for good-tasting products and this is one of their favorites. *Helen & Eric:* Although we didn't think it had a true cheddar taste, it was very flavorful. We ate it plain and also used it to make a delicious turkey melt.
Availability: Supermarkets and health food stores; store locations online

Cheddar, Sharp
Kraft, Cracker Barrel, Reduced Fat, Cheddar Cheese
Kraft Foods, Inc.
800-634-1984 www.kraftfoods.com
Bottom Line: 90 calories per serving (1 oz)
Details: Yummy Hunters cut up and melt thin slices on melba toast for a meal that holds them over for half the day. *Helen:* Very tasty, but if your aim is to get full, you'll be consuming too many calories. I suggest using this as a topping on turkey or veggie burgers. *Eric:* I like to shred some up and put it into an egg-white omelette. Terrific!
Availability: Supermarkets

* Cheddar, Swiss
The Laughing Cow, Light Gourmet, Cheese Bites
Bel/Kaukauna USA, Inc.
920-788-3524 www.thelaughingcow.com
Bottom Line: 35 calories per serving (6 pieces)
Details: One Yummy Hunter takes six pieces with her to work and eats them throughout the day and it keeps her appetite in check. *Helen:* Big taste in every little bite. I like that the consistency is soft enough to spread on a cracker. *Eric:* What an interesting combo. Two of my favorite cheeses in one small package. I used it to make a triple-decker cracker sandwich.
Availability: Supermarkets and ordering online at www.netgrocer.com

* A Low-Fat Product

* Feta
Athenos, Crumbled, Reduced Fat, Feta Cheese
Churny Company, Inc.
800-343-1976 www.athenos.com
Bottom Line: 70 calories per serving (¼ cup)
Details: Yummy Hunters mix it up with some
romaine, some olives; add oil and vinegar and rave
it makes a great Greek salad. *Helen:* We used it to
top a turkey burger and the 1 ounce we spread
added enough taste to make the extra calories
worth it. *Eric:* I love to make feta, tomato and
onion omelettes. A little bit of feta goes a long
way to make a big meal.
Availability: Supermarkets and gourmet shops

* Garlic and Herbs
Boursin, Light, Gournay Cheese Garlic and Herbs
Unilever Best Foods
800-290-5266 www.boursincheese.com
Bottom Line: 39 calories per serving (⅔ tbsp)
Details: Yummy Hunters say they have been eating
the nonlight version and just switched to light and
tell us it's every bit as delicious. *Helen:* We spread
it on a variety of crackers and breads and it was
scrumptious. *Eric:* I can spread this on my hand
and lick my fingers all day, but thanks to Helen I
use crackers. *Helen:* We got him professional help.
Availability: Supermarkets

* Mozzarella
Health Is Wealth, Mozzarella Sticks
Val Vasilef, Health Is Wealth Products, Inc.
856-728-1998 www.healthiswealthfoods.com
Bottom Line: 120 calories per serving (2 sticks)
Details: Yummy Hunters who love mozzarella sticks
can once again enjoy them while dieting. Others
say these are as good as they get in any
restaurant. *Helen:* Everything a good mozzarella
stick should be and more. We dunked them in
Prego's Traditional Pasta Sauce and they were
delicious. *Eric:* Crunchy on the outside, soft and
gooey on the inside. These sticks stick out.
Availability: Supermarkets and health food stores

✳ Mozzarella
Polly-O, Kraft, String – UMS Reduced Fat Mozzarella
Kraft Foods, Inc.
887-476-5596 www.pollyo.com
Bottom Line: 80 calories per serving (1 stick)
Details: Yummy Hunters eat one or two for breakfast and like the fact this delicious product gives them their share of protein. They add it holds them over longer than a bagel. Another Yummy Hunter gives these sticks to her kids and says you can never start early enough when it comes to feeding your family low-fat foods. *Helen & Eric:* So tasty and so much fun to eat.
Availability: Supermarkets

✳ Mozzarella
Polly-O, Light, Shredded Mozzarella
Kraft Foods, Inc.
877-476-5596 www.pollyo.com
Bottom Line: 60 calories per serving (28 g)
Details: Yummy Hunters rave that when they sprinkle this cheese over grilled chicken it makes for an unbelievably tasty meal. Others add it has authentic mozzarella flavor. *Helen & Eric:* It melts so well on everything, whether it's a turkey burger, eggplant or our favorite spinach and mozzarella egg-white omelette.
Availability: Supermarkets

✳ Parmesan
Galaxy Nutritional Foods, Veggy Parmesan
Galaxy Nutritional Foods
407-855-5500 www.galaxyfoods.com
Bottom Line: 15 calories per serving (1 tsp)
Details: Yummy Hunters love it on spaghetti squash and declare it gives the dish a delicious, cheesy flavor. *Helen:* We can't tell the difference between this and Parmesan cheese! *Eric:* A great-tasting cheese to be used anywhere you would use regular Parmesan!
Availability: Health food stores and some supermarkets

Pineapple
Breakstone's, Cottage Doubles, Pineapple
Kraft Foods, Inc.
800-538-1998 www.kraftfoods.com
Bottom Line: 130 calories per serving (1 container)
Details: Yummy Hunters say they take it to work and love to double dip fruit and cottage cheese so they get the right amount in every bite. *Helen & Eric:* The cottage cheese is creamy and delicious and it's nice to have the option of adding as much pineapple as you want.
Availability: Supermarkets

* Swiss
The Laughing Cow, Light, Creamy Swiss
Bel/Kaukauna USA, Inc.
920-788-3524 www.thelaughingcow.com
Bottom Line: 35 calories per serving (1 wedge)
Details: Yummy Hunters say this tasty cheese fills them up and makes them feel like they're eating something fattening. *Helen:* The consistency makes it great for spreading. FYI, one slice is one point on Weight Watchers. *Eric:* The cow's not the only one laughing after you eat this delicious cheese.
Availability: Supermarkets

Have a dieting doubt, spit it out.

CHILI

For us, chili must be thick enough for your spoon to stand straight up and salute you!

---

* Black Bean, Mild
Health Valley, Mild, Black Bean Chili
Hain Celestial Group, Inc.
800-423-4846 www.hain-celestial.com
Bottom Line: 160 calories per serving (1 cup)
Details: Yummy Hunters love the convenience and portability of the can. One Yummy Hunter packs a few when she's traveling and knows she is just a can opener and microwave away from having a delicious meal that keeps her on her diet. *Helen & Eric:* The mild, savory flavor was spicy enough for our palates. It's an extra bonus that this delicious chili is 99 percent fat free and loaded with fiber.
Availability: Supermarkets, health food stores and ordering online at www.leesmarket.com

* Cha-Cha
Fantastic, Cha-Cha Chili, Big Soup Cup
Fantastic Foods, Inc.
800-288-1089 www.fantasticfoods.com
Bottom Line: 220 calories per serving (62 g)
Details: Yummy Hunters who don't eat meat love this veggie delight. They also rave about the convenience. *Helen & Eric:* The container we tried held two servings and not only tasted great but filled us up, too.
Availability: Supermarkets, health food stores and club stores; store locations and ordering online and at www.leesmarket.com

* Chicken, Black Beans
Shelton's, Free Range, Mild, Chicken Chili with Black Beans
Shelton's Poultry, Inc.
800-541-1833 www.sheltons.com
Bottom Line: 210 calories per serving (1 cup)
Details: Yummy Hunters like this hearty, tasty dish and recommend adding low-fat sour cream for a bit of Mexican flair. *Helen:* Because I don't eat meat, this is a very tasty alternative when I'm in the mood for chili. *Eric:* We like the convenience of the can, the chili's robust flavor and the delicious chili — black bean combo.
Availability: Health food stores and online

Chili, Cornbread
Amy's, Chili and Cornbread Whole Meal
Amy's Kitchen, Inc.
707-578-7188 www.amyskitchen.com
Bottom Line: 340 calories per serving (1 meal)
Details: Yummy Hunters say it has just the right amount of spice and rave the corn bread is fluffy and tasty. *Helen:* Hard to believe this deliciously filling meal can be on anyone's diet! *Eric:* This delightful duo creates a satisfying and tasty Mexican meal.
Availability: Health food stores, many supermarkets, some club stores; store locations online and ordering at www.nomeat.com

* Meatless
Boca, Chili, W/Boca Ground Burger
Boca Foods Company
www.bocaburger.com
Bottom Line: 150 calories per serving (269 g)
Details: Yummy Hunters say this stuff is sooo good and loaded with fiber. Another says it's perfect when they don't want to eat a lot of calories for lunch. *Helen:* This full-bodied chili will fill you up, and what a caloric bargain for only 150 calories. *Eric:* I'm chillin' with this chili.
Availability: Supermarkets, health and gourmet food stores; store locations online

* 3-Bean
Fantastic, Fast Naturals Ready Meals, 3-Bean
Fantastic Foods, Inc.
800-288-1089 www.fantasticfoods.com
Bottom Line: 180 calories per serving (227 g)
Details: One Yummy Hunter says she's a vegetarian but her husband isn't; nevertheless, they both love chili and agree this is one tasty dish. Other Yummy Hunters say that when they cook this chili at work all their co-workers want a taste. *Helen:* The spice is right on target. *Eric:* And so are the beans.
Availability: Supermarkets, health food stores and club stores; store locations and ordering online

Vegetable
Amy's, Organic Chili Medium, With Vegetables
Amy's Kitchen, Inc.
707-578-7188 www.amyskitchen.com
Bottom Line: 190 calories per serving (1 cup)
Details: Yummy Hunters love the convenience of this take-along can. They say this is their "when I'm starving meal." *Helen:* Another hit from Amy's. The perfect blend of veggies with just the right bite. *Eric:* Joy to the world, this is for all the boys and girls that love chili.
Availability: Health food stores, many supermarkets, some club stores; store locations online and ordering at www.nomeat.com

Vegetarian
Tabatchnick, Vegetarian Chili
Tabatchnick, Fine Food, Inc.
732-247-6668 www.tabachnick.com
Bottom Line: 180 calories per serving (1 pouch)
Details: Yummy Hunters declare it's easy and delicious. Another complains she's always hungry when she's dieting, but when she eats this chili for lunch, she's happily satisfied. *Helen:* Nice, spicy quality. We agree it's easy, delicious and very filling. *Eric:* I couldn't help myself, I had to crunch up a few Ritz crackers and mix them in.
Availability: Supermarkets

* Vegetarian with Beans
Hormel, Chili Vegetarian with Beans
Hormel Foods Corporation
800-523-4635   www.hormel.com
Bottom Line: 200 calories per serving (1 cup)
Details: One Yummy Hunter sends cans of this chili to her son in college and tells us he and his roommates can't get enough of it. Another says it never goes bad and it's the family's emergency food. *Helen:* Full of spicy goodness and a real hit. *Eric:* Thick and chock full of beans — a vegetarian delight.
Availability: Supermarkets; store locations online

It's still weight from my pregnancy (my son is 20).

CHIPS

Don't tell us that a carrot or celery stick is going to give you the crunch you crave because, until it comes in a plastic bag with salt, that just won't happen. That's why the search for chips was so important— without a great chip there is no way we are ever going on a diet.

―――――――――

Apple
Good Health Crispy Original Apple Chips
Good Health Natural Foods, Inc.
631-261-5608 www.e-goodhealth.com
Bottom Line: 140 calories per serving (12 chips)
Details: Yummy Hunters say it's a dried fruit that crunches like a chip. They love its originality as much as they love the taste. *Helen:* We think they're better than potato chips. *Eric:* So, shoot us!
Availability: Supermarkets, health food stores and online

✳ Barbecue, KC Masterpiece
Baked Lay's Potato Crisps
Frito-Lay, Inc.
800-352-4477 www.fritolay.com
Bottom Line: 120 calories per serving (11 chips)
Details: Yummy Hunters say if they're on a diet, there's no way they're going to serve something they can't eat themselves, so this is their party snack of choice. One Yummy Hunter prefers them to the high-caloric competition because these chips are less greasy. *Helen & Eric:* We layered them on smoked turkey sandwiches and made ourselves a barbecue crunch—yum.
Availability: Supermarkets

* Barbeque, Memphis
Guiltless Gourmet Baked Potato Crisps, Memphis Barbeque
GMB Enterprises, Inc.
800-723-9541 www.guiltlessgourmet.com
Bottom Line: 100 calories per serving (1 oz)
Details: Yummy Hunters love the tangy barbecue flavor. *Helen:* Powerful barbecue flavor that I found very enjoyable. Eric's probably going to say he can't stop eating them. *Eric:* I can't stop eating them!
Availability: Health food stores and some supermarkets; store locations online and ordering at www.leesmarket.com

* Caramel
Glenny's, Low Fat, Soy Crisps, Caramel
Glen Foods, Inc.
888-864-1243 www.glennys.com
Bottom Line: 70 calories per serving (18 g)
Details: Yummy Hunters say that small, portion-controlled bags are always a winner with them. One adds she keeps a bag in her car at all times for hunger emergencies. *Helen:* Glenny's has a way of making delicious low-cal snacks and this one lives up to their great reputation. Tasty, heart-shaped chip with plenty of caramel crunch. *Eric:* A new and very tasty experience.
Availability: Health food stores and some supermarkets; store locations and ordering online

Carrot
Hain Pure Snax Carrot Chips
Hain Celestial Group, Inc.
800-434-4246 www.hainspuresnax.com
Bottom Line: 150 calories per serving (23 chips)
Details: Yummy Hunters find this a great choice for the entire family. They say their kids love 'em without realizing they're getting something good for them. *Helen:* Unique, wheaty taste is combined with a sweet carrot juice flavor. *Eric:* Make a move on this sweet chip.
Availability: Supermarkets and health food stores

✱ Celery
Crispy Delites, 100% Natural Veggie Chips, Celery
Healthy Delite
516-593-5369
Bottom Line: 105 calories per serving (1.07 oz)
Details: Yummy Hunters discovered this new product at their local health food stores and its intriguing flavor led to immediate addiction. They love the strong celery taste and wonderful crunch. *Helen:* For those of you who think crunching a celery stick is boring, wait till you try these babies. *Eric:* Also comes in Asian cucumber and carrot, which are equally spectacular tasting.
Availability: Health food stores

Cheddar
Little Bear, Cheddar Puffs
Hain Celestial Group, Inc.
800-434-4246 www.littlebearfoods.com
Bottom Line: 150 calories per serving (1 cup)
Details: Yummy Hunters measure out their cup and say this is one cheesy snack that seems to last and last and last. *Helen & Eric:* These light cheese puffs explode with flavor.
Availability: Supermarkets and health food stores; ordering online at www.shopnatural.com

✱ Cheddar Cheese, White
Pita Snax Pita Chips, White Cheddar
Pita Products LLC
800-600-7482 www.pitasnax.com
Bottom Line: 120 calories per serving (23 chips)
Details: Yummy Hunters buy the small bags and keep them at their desks. One adds discovering this food gave her the strength to go on with her diet and lose those last 20 difficult pounds. *Helen:* Kudos! My heart goes out to this Yummy Hunter. I know just how difficult her journey was. I just hope the other products in this book can do for others what Pita Snax is doing for her. *Eric:* Amen!
Availability: Supermarkets, health food stores and specialty stores; store locations and ordering online

❋ Cheetos
FritoLay, Baked Cheetos, Crunchy
Frito-Lay, Inc.
800-352-4477 www.fritolay.com
Bottom Line: 130 calories per serving (34 pieces)
Details: Yummy Hunters love the amazing crunch of this cheesy chips. *Helen & Eric:* Bursts of cheesiness in each bite.
Availability: Supermarkets

❋ Chili Cheese
Quaker, Potato Stik, Chili Cheese
The Quaker Oats Company
800-856-5781 www.quakeroats.com
Bottom Line: 110 calories per serving (1 oz)
Details: Yummy Hunters say they love the chili cheese combo. *Helen:* This delicious chip stands on its own. *Eric:* Has a very peppy taste.
Availability: Supermarkets

❋ Corn Chips, Original
Skinny Corn Chips
nSpired Natural Foods
510-686-0116 www.nspiredfoods.com
Bottom Line: 60 calories per serving (1 cup)
Details: Yummy Hunters confess high-calorie chips got them into trouble, but these delicious low-cal chips got them out. *Helen & Eric:* There are corn chips and there are corn chips. These are CORN CHIPS!
Availability: Supermarkets and health food stores; online at www.givemefood.com

❋ Garlic & Chive
Wise, Wise Choice, Roasted Garlic & Chive, Baked Potato Crisps
Wise Foods, Inc.
www.wisesnacks.com
Bottom Line: 110 calories per serving (1¼ cup)
Details: Yummy Hunters rave they have found the ultimate potato chip. *Helen:* Winning combination. *Eric:* Live and eat Chive!
Availability: Health food stores and some supermarkets; store locations online

✱ Mint Fudge
Glenny's Soy Crisps
Glen Foods, Inc.
888-864-1243 www.glennys.com
Bottom Line: 60 calories per serving (about 5 crisps)
Details: Yummy Hunters tell us they get a delicious, chocolatey mint fudge flavor in every bite. They add they couldn't wait to share it with their friends. *Helen:* Spoil the child in you. *Eric:* Get your crunch and sweetness in one deliciously satisfying snack.
Availability: Health food stores and some supermarkets; store locations and ordering online

✱ Mustard & Honey
Kettle Krisps Baked Potato Chips
Kettle Foods
503-364-0399 www.kettlefoods.com
Bottom Line: 110 calories per serving (1 oz)
Details: Yummy Hunters are quick to point out that you better make sure you have someone around when you open a bag; otherwise, you'll be "forced" to eat the whole thing. *Helen:* The perfect potato chip layered with a tasty, honey mustard seasoning on top. *Eric:* For someone who puts mustard on everything, this is a godsend.
Availability: Supermarkets; store locations online and ordering at www.truefoodsmarket.com and www.snackaisle.com

✱ Original
Ritz Chips
Nabisco, Inc.
800-622-4726 www.nabisco.com
Bottom Line: 140 calories per serving (15 chips)
Details: Yummy Hunters say they eat like chips and have that delicious Ritz Cracker taste they've always enjoyed. *Helen:* We ate them plain, then with a little lite cream cheese. *Eric:* Then we did a little song and dance; you guessed it – "Putting on the 'Ritz.'" *Helen:* Sometimes we get carried away.
Availability: Supermarkets

Original
Snapea Crisps
Calbee America, Inc.
310-328-8100
Bottom Line: 150 calories per serving (22 pieces)
Details: Yummy Hunters confess they don't know how these truly innovative chips were made. They rave about the taste, the crunch and the fact the chips are low-carb. *Helen:* One of the most original products we've come across. *Eric:* These green peas that have been magically transformed into chips are one of the most desirable products in this book. These guys should get "The Nobel Eating Prize."
Availability: Supermarkets and health food stores

* Parmesan Garlic & Herb
Stacy's Pita Chips
Stacy's Pita Chip Company, Inc.
888-33-CHIPS www.pitachips.com
Bottom Line: 130 calories per serving (about 8 large chips)
Details: Yummy Hunters rave about their crisp, mouth-watering taste. The use of fresh pita bread leaves a nice, yeasty, wheat taste that is not overpowered by the assertively flavored parmesan-garlic. *Helen:* Our Yummy Hunters say it better than we could. *Eric:* They really are super - delicious.
Availability: Health food stores, some supermarkets and club stores; online at www.givemefood.com and www.leesmarket.com

* Sour Cream & Onion
Glenny's, Spud Delites, Sour Cream & Onion
Glen Foods, Inc.
888-864-1243 www.glennys.com
Bottom Line: 100 calories per serving (1 pckg)
Details: Yummy Hunters say the sour cream and onion flavor makes their mouth water. They say these chips are just terrific. *Helen & Eric:* Low calorie, super crunch, super taste.
Availability: Health food stores and some supermarkets; store locations and ordering online

Sweet Potato
Terra, Sweet Potato Chips
Hain Celestial Group, Inc.
800-434-4246 www.terrachips.com
Bottom Line: 140 calories per serving (1 oz)
Details: Yummy Hunters tell us when they feel the need to indulge in chips these sweet potato chips are so, so satisfying. Another tells us she and her friends open a bag, pass it around at work and that way, no one overdoes it. *Helen:* The perfect chip for sweet potato lovers. Take our Yummy Hunters, advice because once you start eating these, it's hard to stop. *Eric:* Oh, yeah, I'm gonna wait until I have friends around to eat these babies . . . .
Availability: Health food stores and Target Super Stores; store locations online

✱ Vegetable, Original
Pure Snax Crudités Vegetable Snack Twirls
Hain Celestial Group, Inc.
800-434-4246 www.hainspuresnax.com
Bottom Line: 120 calories per serving (30 pieces)
Details: Yummy Hunters proclaim this is one seriously great vegetable chip. Others say they are overjoyed to discover this distinctively delicious snack. *Helen:* This appetizing chip got our attention in a hurry. *Eric:* The skillful combination of flavors is only outdone by the crunchy vegetable goodness.
Availability: Supermarkets and health food stores

✱ Veggies
Just Veggies
Just Tomatoes
209-894-5371 www.justtomatoes.com
Bottom Line: 100 calories per serving (1 oz)
Details: Yummy Hunters tell us they eat them right out of the container. They also add them to their favorite soups. *Helen & Eric:* Crunches like popcorn, tastes like veggies and is another one of the brilliantly unique creations our Yummy Hunters have discovered.
Availability: Health food stores and online

✳ White Cheddar
Stacy's Thin Crisps, Baked Soy Chips
Stacy's Pita Chip Company, Inc.
888-33-CHIPS www.pitachip.com
Bottom Line: 106 calories per serving (25 crisps)
Details: Yummy Hunters eat them with lunch, as snacks or just nosh on them all day long. They add it has just the right amount of white cheddar seasoning. *Helen & Eric:* Zesty, tangy and kicking good.
Availability: Health food stores, some supermarkets and club stores; ordering online at www.givemefood.com

✳ Yellow Corn
Guiltless Gourmet Baked Tortilla Chips
GMB Enterprises, Inc.
800-723-9541 www.guiltlessgourmet.com
Bottom Line: 110 calories per serving (1 oz or 18 chips)
Details: Yummy Hunters say they love these hearty, baked corn chips. They add the chips have a strong corn flavor, which adds to their sweet taste. Others add they're great for dipping into chunky salsa because they don't fall apart. *Helen:* One mighty strong and fine corn chip! *Eric:* We dipped them into salsa and then into Mrs. Renfro's Cheese Sauce and they were delicious.
Availability: Health food stores and some supermarkets; store locations online and ordering at www.leesmarket.com

Yogurt and Green Onion
Barbara's, Potato Chips, Yogurt and Green Onion
Barbara's For A Brighter Future
707-765-2273 www.barbarasbakery.com
Bottom Line: 150 calories per serving (1¼ cup)
Details: Yummy Hunters who love potato chips can't wait to share this new discovery with like-minded fans. *Helen:* The yogurt and onion flavors pair up perfectly . *Eric:* Wowie!
Availability: Health food stores and some supermarkets; store locations online

Zesty Tomato
Terra Vegetable Chips
Hain Celestial Group, Inc.
800-434-4246 www.terrachips.com
Bottom Line: 140 calories per serving (10 pieces)
Details: One Yummy Hunter lamented these chips are so good, they're "evil." Another said if he didn't watch himself, he would eat the whole bag at one sitting. *Helen:* Infused with tangy, tomato flavor. *Eric:* They're delicious; mighty risky if you don't know when to say when.
Availability: Health food stores and Target Super Stores; store locations online

I keep trying to lose weight, but it keeps finding me.

CONDIMENTS
MAYONNAISE, MUSTARD, ONIONS, PEPPERS, PICKLES, SALSA, STEAK SAUCES

WE ALL RELISH a delicious condiment — otherwise, our diets are in a pickle.

MAYONNAISE

* Chipotle Chili
French's, GourMayo, Chipotle Chili
French's Foodservice
800-442-4733 www.frenchsfoodservice.com
Bottom Line: 50 calories per serving (1 tsp)
Details: Yummy Hunters spread a little over light cheese or between slices of light bread. *Helen:* Add it to a turkey sandwich for a south-of-the-border flavor. *Eric:* French's also makes this GourMayo in Sun Dried Tomato and Wasabi Horseradish flavors. Say goodbye to mayonnaise, say hello to GourMayo!
Availability: Supermarkets

* Light
Hellmann's, Light Mayonnaise
Unilever Best Foods
800-838-8831 www.mayo.com
Bottom Line: 45 calories per serving (1 tbsp)
Details: Yummy Hunters couldn't believe the flavor of Hellmann's Light. They put it on sandwiches, mix it into tuna salads and won't go back to regular mayo. *Helen:* We made chicken salad. Delish! *Eric:* We even mixed it with a little ketchup and made a tasty Russian veggie dip.
Availability: Supermarkets

MUSTARD

✳ Apricot Ginger
Robert Rothschild, Apricot Ginger Mustard
Robert Rothschild Berry Farm, Inc.
800-356-8933 www.robertrothschild.com
Bottom Line: 20 calories per serving (1 tbsp)
Details: Yummy Hunters used to use this as a glaze for ham, but now that they're dieting they use it on roasted chicken breasts. Mixed with light mayo it also makes a delicious salad dressing. *Helen & Eric:* First, we licked it off our fingers, then we actually used the product as intended and we rolled up some turkey and dipped it. Oh boy, oh boy!
Availability: Gourmet shops; store locations and ordering online and at www.gourmetcountry.com

✳ Brown Mustard
Eden Organic, Brown Mustard
Eden Foods, Inc.
 www.edenfoods.com
Bottom Line: 0 calories per serving (1 tsp)
Details: Yummy Hunters who are mustard happy say this is one tasty mustard. When dieting, mustard is a great condiment because it adds flavor without adding calories. *Helen & Eric:* We spread it on top of a piece of salmon, broiled the fish and it made for a great meal.
Availability: Health food stores and online

✳ Country Dijon
Grey Poupon, Country Dijon Mustard
Nabisco, Inc.
800-622-1726 www.nabisco.com
Bottom Line: 5 calories per serving (1 tsp)
Details: Yummy Hunters say this is the great spicy mustard they use instead of mayo on turkey sandwiches. Others tell us it perks up their hot dogs and is a must-dip on pretzels. *Helen:* The dipping thing is a must for dieters, so I dip my pretzel to our Yummy Hunters. *Eric:* Hot stuff, any way you look at it!
Availability: Supermarkets

✳ A Low-Fat Product

✳ Raspberry
Annie's Naturals, Organic Raspberry Mustard
Annie's Naturals
800-434-1234 www.anniesnaturals.com
Bottom Line: 5 calories per serving (1 tsp)
Details: Yummy Hunters say the fruit flavor combined with the mustard makes for one really unique and delicious taste. *Helen:* We spread it on turkey and it gave the meat a special sweet-and-sour flavor. *Eric:* Spread it around, this is one delicious mustard.
Availability: Supermarkets, health food stores and chains

ONIONS

✳ Onion
Sabrett, Onions in Sauce
Marathon Enterprises, Inc.
800-468-3646 www.sabrett.com
Bottom Line: 10 calories per serving (1 tbsp)
Details: Yummy Hunters put it on a low-fat hotdog, and they say it's got so much flavor they don't need mustard. *Helen:* They really bring out the flavor of turkey burgers. *Eric:* I put 'em on dogs and burgers and don't tell anyone about this . . . sometimes by themselves on a bun.
Availability: Supermarkets, wholesale clubs and online at www.foodsofnewyork.com

PEPPERS

✳ Hot Cherry Peppers
Haddon House, Hoagie Spread Hot Cherry Peppers
Haddon House Food Products
800-257-6174 www.haddonhouse.com
Bottom Line: 5 calories per serving (1 tbsp)
Details: Yummy Hunters spread a little on a turkey sandwich and it really provides unique spicy taste. *Helen & Eric:* We made turkey sandwiches, put on the hoagie spread and some fat-free Russian dressing and it was so hot it was cool!
Availability: Supermarkets

* Pepper
Vlasic, Pepper Stackers
Pinnacle Foods Corporation
800-421-3265 www.vlasic.com
Bottom Line: 5 calories per serving (12 rings)
Details: Yummy Hunters say when dieting, cold cuts on low-fat bread are a staple. Adding Vlasic Pepper Stackers transforms sandwiches into new and exciting meals. *Helen:* For variety try these peppers on low-fat cheese. *Eric:* Since childhood I've loved to stack pickles. Stacking peppers is a new and exciting treat for me.
Availability: Supermarkets

* Roasted
B&G, Roasted Red Peppers
B&G Foods, Inc.
www.bgfoods.com
Bottom Line: 10 calories per serving (½ pepper)
Details: Yummy Hunters can eat the entire jar and not feel guilty. Others add these peppers spice up bag lunches that they take to work. *Helen:* When I have company, I make a chopped salad, put roasted red peppers and light mozzarella on top and add Cardini's Fat Free Caesar. I get rave reviews all the time. *Eric:* She's such a gourmet.
Availability: Supermarkets, by phone and ordering online at www.mybrandsinc.com

* Roasted
Victoria, Red Roasted Peppers
Victoria Packing Corp.
718-927-3000 www.victoriapacking.com
Bottom Line: 24 calories per serving (⅓ cup)
Details: Yummy Hunters say they like to get the most volume out of each food, and these red roasted peppers really help. Yummy Hunters add them to egg-white omelettes. *Helen & Eric:* Another great pepper option. One day, we'll combine all their selections and pepper out!
Availability: Supermarkets and ordering online at www.newyorkflavors.com

PICKLES

✳ Dill
Vlasic, Baby Kosher Dills
Pinnacle Foods Corporation
800-421-3265 www.vlasic.com
Bottom Line: 5 calories per serving (1 oz)
Details: Yummy Hunters say they're delicious and fill their craving for salt and something crunchy. *Helen:* They're salty, crunchy and we eat 'em to our hearts' content; however, if you're worried about water retention, too many can put you into a different kind of pickle. *Eric:* These babies have a grown-up taste.
Availability: Supermarkets

✳ Dill
Vlasic, Oval Hamburger Dill Chips
Pinnacle Foods Corporation
800-421-3265 www.vlasic.com
Bottom Line: 5 calories per serving (3 slices)
Details: Yummy Hunters rave about how everyone in the family loves to put them on everything from hamburgers to tuna fish sandwiches. *Helen:* Tastes just like dill deli pickles. Yummy! *Eric:* You never want to run out of these delicious chips. If I could find a reason to eat them at breakfast, I would.
Availability: Supermarkets

✳ Dill
Vlasic, Snack'MMS
Pinnacle Foods Corporation
800-421-3265 www.vlasic.com
Bottom Line: 5 calories per serving (2 pickles)
Details: Yummy Hunters who love dill pickles keep a jar around for a 5-calorie crunch. *Helen:* Great for sprucing up salads. This is one cute, mouth-watering crunch. *Eric:* Who in their right mind takes the time to actually see if these pickles are cute? I say, open the jar and get 'em into your mouth or on a sandwich as fast as you can!
Availability: Supermarkets

* Kosher Dill
Claussen, Kosher Dill Halves
Kraft Foods, Inc.
800-322-1421 www.kraft.com
Bottom Line: 5 calories per serving (½ pickle)
Details: Yummy Hunters rave this is truly the best pickle on the market. One says when all her pickles are gone, she slices a cucumber and puts it into the remaining liquid and — presto! — twenty-four hours later she has half-sour pickles. *Helen:* That Yummy Hunter sure knows how to get the most from her pickle purchase. *Eric:* First time I ever heard of someone getting out of a pickle by getting into one.
Availability: Supermarkets

SALSA

* Artichoke
Santa Barbara, Artichoke
California Creative Foods, Inc.
800-748-5523 www.sbsalsa.com
Bottom Line: 15 calories per serving (2 tbsp)
Details: One Yummy Hunter said this was the best salsa she ever had. *Helen:* We love artichokes and we love this salsa. *Eric:* This is the first time I ever had artichokes and salsa and it was terrific.
Availability: Supermarkets and online

* Black Bean & Corn
Amy's, Organic Salsa
Amy's Kitchen, Inc.
707-578-7188 www.amyskitchen.com
Bottom Line: 15 calories per serving (2 tbsp)
Details: One Yummy Hunter tells us she makes eggs for lunch and adds this salsa for a real Mexican treat. *Helen:* Corn and black bean add a special flare to this tasty salsa. *Eric:* Sweet!
Availability: Health food stores, many supermarkets, some club stores; store locations online and ordering at www.nomeat.com

✳ Black Bean & Corn
Santa Barbara, Black Bean & Corn
California Creative Foods, Inc.
800-748-5523 www.sbsalsa.com
Bottom Line: 15 calories per serving (2 tbsp)
Details: One Yummy Hunter said this is one addictive salsa. *Helen:* The black beans add a thick consistency to this special salsa. *Eric:* Another sweet-tasting salsa.
Availability: Supermarkets and online

✳ Salsa, Mild
Green Mountain Gringo, Mild Salsa
Green Mountain Gringo
888-875-3111 www.greenmountaingringo.com
Bottom Line: 10 calories per serving (2 tbsp)
Details: When Yummy Hunters watch TV, instead of high-calorie snacks, they break out the Skinny Chips and the Green Mountain. *Helen:* We dipped peppers and cucumbers and came up for air when the plate was empty. *Eric:* I put it on everything. Thank God I have willpower or I would brush with it. Comes in medium and hot, for all you flame-thrower types.
Availability: Most health food stores, some supermarkets, online and at www.leesmarket.com

✳ Salsa, Mild
Tostitos, Mild Salsa
Frito-Lay, Inc.
800-352-4477 www.tostitos.com
Bottom Line: 15 calories per serving (2 tbsp)
Details: One Yummy Hunter jokes that when dieting she salsas everything—sandwiches, salads, tacos and even her husband. *Helen:* This is one salsa-crazy Yummy Hunter, but we know how salsa can brighten up almost everything, so all we can say is, go, girl, go. *Eric:* Yummy Hunters all like the medium and hot versions, but we won't go there without more medical coverage.
Availability: Supermarkets and ordering online at www.leesmarket.com

✳ Salsa, Southwestern
Guiltless Gourmet, Southwestern Grill Salsa, Fat Free
GMB Enterprises, Inc.
800-723-9541 www.guiltlessgourmet.com
Bottom Line: 15 calories per serving (2 tbsp)
Details: One Yummy Hunter tells us when she serves this her guests clamor for the recipe and when she tells them it was store-bought, they don't believe it. Others rave it has the smoky barbeque flavor they love. *Helen & Eric:* It tastes just like it was cooked on a backyard barbeque.
Availability: Supermarkets and health food stores

STEAK SAUCES

✳ Steak House
Peter Luger, Steak House Old Fashioned Steak Sauce
Peter Luger Enterprises, Inc.
718-387-0500 www.peterluger.com
Bottom Line: 30 calories per serving (1 tbsp)
Details: Yummy Hunters use it on steaks and as a marinade for chicken. *Helen:* We followed the company's serving suggestions from the website, mixing low-fat mayo with the sauce, to make the best Russian dressing we ever had. *Eric:* This will have to hold me until I make it to Peter Luger's — which I hope will be this year.
Availability: Supermarkets in New York, New Jersey, Florida, by phone and online

✳ Steak Sauce
A1, Steak Sauce
Kraft Foods, Inc.
800-538-1998 www.kraftfoods.com
Bottom Line: 15 calories per serving (1 tbsp)
Details: Yummy Hunters proclaim they've been eating A1 since childhood, so when they allow themselves a piece of steak, it's never complete without A1. *Helen:* This sauce is great on chicken and turkey. *Eric:* And on steak, veal and, yes — hot dogs!
Availability: Supermarkets and ordering online at www.netgrocer.com

* Steak Sauce

KC Masterpiece, Original, Steakhouse, Barbecue Sauce

The HV Food Products Company
800-537-2823 www.kcmasterpiece.com
Bottom Line: 60 calories per serving (2 tbsp)
Details: Yummy Hunters who need their meat tell us this is their favorite barbecue sauce. They add that a steak just isn't a steak unless they use KC Masterpiece steak sauce. *Helen:* Oh, this is really good! *Eric:* While Helen's totally overcome with rapture, let me say we had it on chicken and it gave it a mouth-watering, backyard-barbecue flavor.
Availability: Supermarkets and discount stores

Dieting is wishful shrinking.

COOKIES

BROWNIES, COOKIES

A COOKIE inspired Helen to write this book. Coincidence? I think not! The great Food Goddess In The Sky knows how addicted she is to those crunchy beauties and wanted her to share her knowledge with others like her. Thank you, oh Food Goddess!

BROWNIES

* Fudge
No Pudge Original Fudge Brownie Mix
No Pudge Foods, Inc.
800-667-8343 www.nopudge.com
Bottom Line: 110 calories per serving dry mix (¹⁄₁₂ pckg)
Details: Yummy Hunters following Weight Watchers scream with delight over these delicious 2-point-per-serving brownies. The smell of fresh-baked brownies inspires them to stay focused on their diet all day long. *Helen:* I needed 6 points to satisfy my chocolate cravings. *Eric:* Rich, gooey and chocolatey, plus you gotta love the name.
Availability: Supermarkets and online

COOKIES

* Alphabet
Newman's Own Organics, Alphabet Cookies
Newman's Own Organics, The Second Generation
www.newmansownorganics.com
Bottom Line: 120 calories per serving (10 cookies)
Details: Yummy Hunters say they taste just like animal crackers. *Helen:* First, we spelled out our names, and then we gobbled down these delicious cookies. *Eric:* We applaud the fact all profits go to educational and charitable purposes.
Availability: Supermarkets and health food stores; store locations online

* Animal Crackers
Nabisco, Barnum's, Animal Crackers
Nabisco, Inc.
800-Nabisco www.nabiscoworld.com
Bottom Line: 130 calories per serving (10 crackers)
Details: One Yummy Hunter says it's the family favorite. Another says she has no guilt when her family gobbles them up. *Helen:* They may call it a cracker, but it's a cookie to me and tastes just as good as it did when I was a child! *Eric:* Uniquely sweet and tasty.
Availability: Supermarkets

* Anisette Toast
Stella D'Oro, Anisette Toast Cookies
Kraft Foods, Inc.
888-878-3552 www.kraftfoods.com
Bottom Line: 130 calories per serving (3 cookies)
Details: Yummy Hunters declare when they have these with coffee, they feel like they're in a European bistro! *Helen & Eric:* An old-time favorite. If ya got 'em—dunk 'em!
Availability: Some supermarkets; phone for store locations and online at www.netgrocer.com

* Apple Pie
Immaculate Baking Co., Apple Pie, Apple Crumble
Immaculate Baking Company
828-696-1655 www.immaculatebaking.com
Bottom Line: 110 calories per serving (4 cookies)
Details: Yummy Hunters rate them number one on their cookie list. They crumple a few and put them on top of low-fat ice cream and rave about how unbelievably delicious it is. *Helen:* Oh, man, are they delicious! We could have had the entire box at one sitting, but thank goodness we are reasonable people and saw the error of our ways before it was too late. *Eric:* What she means is, we were down to the crumbs, so we figured we might as well stop. We admire the fact that the company donates 5 percent of all profits to the Folk Art Foundation.
Availability: Some health food stores; store locations and ordering online

* Black and White
Nutritious Creations, Sugar Free, Black & White
Nutritious Creations, LTD
631-666-9815 www.bakedgoods.tv
Bottom Line: 107 calories per serving (½ cookie)
Details: Yummy Hunters who have a fondness for black, and, white cookies rate these right up at the top. They add,they taste bakery fresh. *Helen:* Super cookie with a sweet top. I break it in two and it gets me through an entire afternoon. *Eric:* As big as a flying saucer. From licking the chocolate top to savoring the cake-like bottom, this is so sweet.
Availability: Health food stores, delis and online

* Black Forest
Snackwell's Cookie Cakes, Black Forest
Kraft Foods, Inc.
800-622-4726 www.nabiscoworld.com
Bottom Line: 50 calories per serving (1 cookie)
Details: One Yummy Hunter told us she has been following a low-fat diet for the past six months and these cookies have helped her control her cravings for sweets. She has lost 38 pounds so far and claims these delicious new cookies were heaven sent. *Helen:* A thin layer of marshmallow covers this moist cake-like cookie. If that's not enough to tempt you, the entire thing is covered with chocolate. *Eric:* Into the black forest we go, we go.
Availability: Supermarkets

* Chocolate
The Smarter Carb, Chocolate-Covered Meringues
BP Gourmet, LTD
631-234-5200 www.bpgourmet.com
Bottom Line: 90 calories per serving (6 cookies)
Details: Yummy Hunters rave how chocolatey and crunchy these delicious cookies are to eat and eat and eat. *Helen & Eric:* Therein lies the problem. Buyers beware—keep to the serving size or else, or else, or else.
Availability: Supermarkets and health food stores

* Chocolate Chip
Entenmann's, Chewy Chocolate Chip Cookies
A Unit of George Weston Bakeries, Inc.
800-356-3314 www.gwbakeries.com
Bottom Line: 130 calories per serving (3 cookies)
Details: Yummy Hunters say they wouldn't buy another brand. Entenmann's has been a family favorite for generations. *Helen:* Really soft and chewy and oh, so, full of chocolate chips. *Eric:* Warning, warning, warning! Eat at your own risk! Now if I could only follow my own advice.
Availability: Sporadic throughout the United States and ordering online at www.netgrocer.com

* Chocolate Chip
Rising Dough, Chocolate Chip Cookie
Rising Dough Bakery
877-349-8900 www.risingdough.com
Bottom Line: 90 calories per serving (1½ oz)
Details: Yummy Hunters tell us that right out of the package it's soft and chewy and satisfying. *Helen:* My dieting daughter loves these so much, I order them online by the box. It's a full-sized cookie that holds her over for the day. *Eric:* Can't wait until they speed up the Internet and these cookies come right out of my computer. Available in oatmeal chocolate chip, so knock yourself out.
Availability: Online

* Chocolate Chip
The Smarter Carb, Chocolate Chip Biscotti
BP Gourmet, LTD
631-234-5200 www.bpgourmet.com
Bottom Line: 50 calories per serving (3 cookies)
Details: Yummy Hunters say they have an almond taste that mixes well with the chocolate. They add their kids love them with ice cream. *Helen & Eric:* The company calls its product "the diet treat with premium taste", otherwise, that's what we would have said.
Availability: Online at www.gethealthyamerica.com and www.leesmarket.com

Chocolate Chip With Pecans
Joseph's, Sugar-Free Cookies, Chocolate Chip With Pecans
Joseph's Lite Cookies
505-546-2839 www.josephslitecookies.com
Bottom Line: 95 calories per serving (4 cookies)
Details: Yummy Hunters rave what fattening-tasting cookies these are. *Helen & Eric:* The pecans make this special cookie even more special.
Availability: Supermarkets, health food stores, ordering online and at www.givemefood.com and www.netgrocer.com

Chocolate Raspberry
Joseph's, Sugar-Free Cake, Chocolate Raspberry
Joseph's Lite Cookies
505-546-2839 www.josephslitecookies.com
Bottom Line: 100 calories per serving (4 cakes)
Details: Yummy Hunters say these raspberry treats break up a hum-drum afternoon. *Helen:* Tasty cookie with the perfect amount of raspberry sweetness. *Eric:* So small, but so good.
Availability: Supermarkets, health food stores, online and ordering at www.givemefood.com and www.netgrocer.om

* Cinnamon
Barbara's, Organic Go Go Grahams, Cinnamon
Barbara's Bakery, Inc.
707-765-2273 www.barbarasbakery.com
Bottom Line: 130 calories per serving (8 cookies)
Details: Yummy Hunters say they're light and crispy and just melt in their mouth. They dunk them in low-fat milk and feel like a little kid again. *Helen:* Outstanding cinnamon flavor and the crisp consistency make them dangerously good. I just wish instead of making me feel like a kid, they made me look like one again. *Eric:* Yum Yum at the Go Go! They also come in chocolate flavor.
Availability: Supermarkets and health food stores; store locations online and ordering at www.leesmarket.com and www.truefoodsmarket

* Cinnamon Raisin
Health Valley, Fat Free, Cinnamon Raisin, Scones
Hain Celestial Group, Inc.
800-423-4846 www.hain-celestial.com
Bottom Line: 180 calories per serving (1 scone)
Details: Yummy Hunters say these scones remind them of their childhood and chirp how nice it is to diet with an old favorite. *Helen:* They make a quick and easy breakfast or a filling in-between snack. *Eric:* So good, these scones will gather no moss.
Availability: Supermarkets, health food stores and ordering online at www.leesmarket.com, www.naturemart.com and www.netgrocer.com

* Cranberry
THIN Addictives, Cranberry Almond Thins
Thin Addictives
888-667-6669 www.thinaddictives.com
Bottom Line: 90 calories per serving (3 cookies)
Details: Yummy Hunters say these cookies are thin and sweet and they like the fact that they come prepackaged. *Helen:* These thin, crunchy biscuits loaded with cranberries, almonds and raisins are an absolute must-try. *Eric:* We just kept opening packages and lost count. I suggest you have a calculator at your elbow or a friend who will count out loud the number of cookies you've eaten. Hopefully, he will also have the courage to pull the pack away from you when you have reached your quota.
Availability: Supermarkets and club stores

* Double Chocolate Chip
Rising Dough, Double, Chocolate Chip Cookie
Rising Dough Bakery
877-349-8900 www.risingdough.com
Bottom Line: 100 calories per serving (1½ oz)
Details: Yummy Hunters tell us that never in their lives have they had such a delicious chocolate experience. *Helen:* A chocolate lover's dream. *Eric:* The stuff dreams are made of.
Availability: Online

* Fig

Nabisco, Fat-Free Fig Newtons

Nabisco, Inc.

800-Nabisco www.nabiscoworld.com

Bottom Line: 100 calories per serving (2 Newtons)

Details: Yummy Hunters have loved these since childhood. They add the familiar fruity taste is a comfort. One says, "I am not a chocolate person; however, I have just as much of a sweet tooth and these Newtons satisfy my cravings." *Helen:* A timeless classic, and we think, in moderation, it fits into any low-calorie diet plan. *Eric:* Great fig flavor. So, were Newtons named after Sir Isaac Newton?

Available: Supermarkets

Fudge Dipped, Graham Crackers

Murray, Sugar Free, Fudge Dipped, Graham

Murray Biscuit Company

877-745-5582 www.murraysugarfree.com

Bottom Line: 130 calories per serving (5 cookies)

Details: One Yummy Hunter said these are as good as her childhood favorites. Another says she really likes the rich chocolate coating on the crispy graham cracker. *Helen:* Chocolate-covered grahams at their best. *Eric:* Murray does it again.

Availability: Supermarkets and drugstores

Fudge Dipped, Short Bread

Murray, Sugar Free, Fudge Dipped, Short Bread Cookies

Murray Biscuit Company

877-745-5582 www.murraysugarfree.com

Bottom Line: 130 calories per serving (5 cookies)

Details: One Yummy Hunter makes a cup of coffee and has two of these cookies every night. The sweetness of these treats is enough to satisfy her sweet tooth and helped her to stay with her diet plan. Subsequently, she lost 30 pounds. *Helen:* I'm so proud of her! *Eric:* Hey, Murray, who taught you to make such delicious fudge-dipped cookies?

Availability: Supermarkets and drugstores

* Lemon White Chocolate Chip
Immaculate Baking Co., Leapin' Lemon, Lemon White Chocolate Chip
Immaculate Baking Company
828-696-1655 www.immaculatebaking.com
Bottom Line: 150 calories per serving (5 cookies)
Details: *Helen:* I could easily eat the entire package, that's how good these are. *Eric:* Always carry one in case you spot Elvis, at which time you will give him one and in return he will appear with you on *Oprah. Helen:* They're that good!
Availability: Some health food stores; store locations and ordering online

Oatmeal
Joseph's, Oatmeal, Sugar Free Cookies
Joseph's Lite Cookies
505-546-2839 www.josephslitecookies.com
Bottom Line: 100 calories per serving (4 cookies)
Details: Yummy Hunters have one word for these cookies — sensational! They eat them for snacks, with coffee and always put them out for company. *Helen:* Sweet, crunchy oatmeal cookie. As soon as we run out, my kids beg for more. *Eric:* Who said beggars aren't choosers?
Availability: Health food stores, some supermarkets, online and at www.givemefood.com and www.netgrocer.com

* Oatmeal Cranberry Raisin
Rising Dough, Oatmeal, Cranberry Raisin Cookie
Rising Dough Bakery
877-349-8900 www.risingdough.com
Bottom Line: 70 calories per serving (1½ oz)
Details: Yummy Hunters discovered this oatmeal cookie online and say this delicious cookie is a sweet alternative to the traditional raisin cookie. *Helen:* Dry cranberries add sweetness to this oatmeal raisin delight. *Eric:* Rising Dough rises to the top with this chewy, fruity gem that is indescribably delicious.
Availability: Online

✳ Orange
Aunt Gussie's, No Sugar Added, Orange Biscottini
Aunt Gussie's Cookies and Crackers
880-4-A-Cookie www.auntgussies.com
Bottom Line: 100 calories per serving (5 cookies)
Details: Yummy Hunters serve these Aunt Gussie's biscottini at monthly book club meetings and tell us they're great for dunking. *Helen & Eric:* The orange spice makes this a delicious complement to flavored teas.
Availability: Health food stores; store locations and ordering online

✳ Potato Chip
Immaculate Baking Co., Potato Chip Cookies, Sweet And Salty Shortbread
Immaculate Baking Company
828-696-1655 www.immaculatebaking.com
Bottom Line: 140 calories per serving (4 cookies)
Details: *Helen*: The battle between salty and sweet releases the ultimate taste sensation as you bite down on these delicious cookies. Tastes like a potato chip! *Eric:* Always carry one in case you meet that teacher who never thought you would amount to anything, at which point you will offer her a cookie and watch as she falls to her knees asking you to forgive her.
Availability: Some health food stores; store locations and ordering online

✳ Raisin Oatmeal
Health Valley, Fat Free, Raisin Oatmeal Cookies
Hain Celestial Group, Inc.
800-423-4846 www.hain-celestial.com
Bottom Line: 100 calories per serving (3 cookies)
Details: Yummy Hunters tell us they love cookies but cookies don't love them—until now when they've finally found a delicious low-cal favorite that won't do them in. *Helen:* I hear you! *Eric:* Big raisin oatmeal taste. Really, really good.
Availability: Supermarkets, health food stores, and online at www.leesmarket.com, www.naturemart.com and www.netgrocer.com

Triple Chocolate Chunk
Immaculate Baking Co., Sweet Georgia Brownie, Triple Chocolate Chunk
Immaculate Baking Company
828-696-1655 www.immaculatebaking.com
Bottom Line: 130 calories per serving (5 cookies)
Details: *Helen:* These knocked my socks off. *Eric:* Always carry one for those times you wonder why you are here and what the purpose of life is.
Availability: Some health food stores; store locations and ordering online

* Vanilla
Heavenly Desserts, Sugar Free, Fat Free Meringue, Vanilla
D-Liteful Bakery, Inc.
www.heavenlydessert.com
Bottom Line: 12 calories per serving (3 cookies)
Details: Yummy Hunters say they are so good, they have to be bad for you! Sweet and crunchy, they can eat these cookies all day without guilt! *Helen:* This is the cookie that inspired me to write this book. The calorie count has changed, so I'm sorry to say this cookie is now 4 calories instead of 0. I can still live with that. *Eric:* Me, too!
Availability: Online at www.gethealthyamerica.com

* Wild Raspberry
Barry's Bakery, French Twists, Wild Raspberry
Barry's Bakery
800-894-7887 www.barrysbakery.com
Bottom Line: 60 calories per serving (1 twist)
Details: Yummy Hunters rave about these crunchy pastry puffs. They say these taste like the most fattening French pastry and can't believe the twists contain no butter. Others recommend the Maple French Toast and Chocolate Chip flavors. *Helen & Eric:* This is one looooong and delicious twist!
Availability: Supermarkets and delis; ordering online and at www.amazon.com

A balanced diet is a cookie in each hand.

* A Low-Fat Product

CRACKERS

Crackers, Rice Cakes

Crunch 'em, munch 'em, eat 'em by the bunch
'em! And no cracks, dieters, you know
no diet works without 'em.

CRACKERS

* Bran
**FiberRich, 100% Natural Wheat Brand, Fiber
Crackers**
Saetre AS
www.lowcarbnexus.com
Bottom Line: 35 calories per serving (2 crackers)
Details: Yummy Hunters love them because the
carb count is so low and the fiber count's so high.
They use them instead of bread with some low-fat
cheese or tuna. *Helen & Eric:* We tried the Yummy
Hunters' suggestions and it was everything they
said; however, when eaten plain, we found these
crackers to be a little bland for our palates.
Availability: Online

* Brown Rice
Hol Grain Crackers, No Salt, Brown Rice
Conrad Rice Mills, Inc.
www.holgrain.com
Bottom Line: 60 calories per serving (7 crackers)
Details: Yummy Hunters who have to watch their
sodium intake tell us these crackers are light and
delicious right out of the bag or with a smear of
cream cheese. *Helen:* It's amazing that just one
ingredient — ice — can have so much taste. *Eric:* It's
not for us to question, only for us to eat.
Availability: Health food stores and online

Cheese
Nabisco 100 Calorie Packs, Kraft, Cheese Nips, Thin Crisps
Nabisco, Inc.
800-622-4726 www.nabiscoworld.com
Bottom Line: 100 calories per serving (1 pack)
Details: Yummy Hunters who need to measure out portions love the convenience. They also rave about the rich cheese taste. *Helen:* The right amount of calories with more than the right amount of deliciousness. *Eric:* These tasty little wonders will nip any hunger pangs in the bud and, best of all, won't leave any cheesy residue that you can't take care of with one quick lick.
 Availability: Supermarkets

✱ Garlic
Devonsheer, Mini Bagel Snacks, Garlic
Old London Foods, Inc.
718-409-1776 www.oldlondonmelba.com
Bottom Line: 50 calories per serving (8 pieces)
Details: Bagel-loving Yummy Hunters say these taste like mini toasted bagels. *Helen:* They reminded us of the bagel crisps we get at the bagel store. *Eric:* We made mini pizza bagels and they were mini, mini good.
Availability: Some supermarkets and ordering online at www.truefoodsmarket.com

MultiGrain
Wasa, MultiGrain, Crisp Bread
Wasa North America
www.wasa-usa.com
Bottom Line: 40 calories per serving (1 cracker)
Details: Yummy Hunters tell us when they want a thicker, more filling cracker this is their pick. *Helen:* I agree with our Yummy Hunters. Great by itself or with a smear of cream cheese. *Eric:* I like the rich, hearty flavor and especially like to spread some Brummel & Brown on top. Always makes for a satisfying in-between meal snack.
Availability: Supermarkets, gourmet shops, online

✱ Original
Ritz Chips
Nabisco, Inc.
800-622-4726 www.nabisco.com
Bottom Line: 140 calories per serving (15 chips)
Details: Yummy Hunters say these eat like chips and have that delicious Ritz Cracker taste they've always enjoyed. *Helen:* We ate them plain, then with a little lite cream cheese. *Eric:* "Putting on the 'Ritz.'" *Helen:* Sometimes we get carried away.
Availability: Supermarkets

✱ Original 7 Grain
Kashi, TLC, Original 7 Grain
Kashi Company
858-274-8870 www.kashi.com
Bottom Line: 130 calories per serving (15 crackers)
Details: Yummy Hunters unequivocally praise these as the best crackers they've ever had. One said she's on Weight Watchers, so she measures out 2 points worth and then takes them to work and can't wait until snack time. *Helen:* The ultimate complement, we ate them right out of the box. *Eric:* Give them plenty of TLC; these TLC crackers are tender-loving good.
Availability: Supermarkets

✱ Pecan
Blue Diamond, Nut-Thins, Pecan
Blue Diamond Growers
916-442-0777 www.bluediamond.com
Bottom Line: 130 calories per serving (16 crackers)
Details: Yummy Hunters say these crackers have a very natural, nutty flavor. They love to eat them with tuna fish salad. *Helen:* A compelling cracker that adds a special nutty crunch to all your favorite cheeses and spreads. *Eric:* A snack in and of itself. Beats me how they can get so much flavor and crunchiness into one thin cracker.
Availability: Supermarkets, health food stores, online and ordering at www.leesmarket.com and truefoodsmarket.com

* Pretzel
The Snack Factory, Pretzel Crisps
The Snack Factory
609-683-5400 www.pretzelcrisps.com
Bottom Line: 110 calories per serving (20 crisps)
Details: One Yummy Hunter says the flat surface holds the perfect amount of any kind of spread. *Helen:* Nice texture and great taste. A uniquely creative product. *Eric:* Be the first on your block to make a triple-decker cracker/pretzel sandwich. I put Brummel & Brown Yogurt on the bottom and a piece of low-fat cheese on the top.
Availability: Supermarkets

* Roasted Garlic and Rosemary
Partners, Low Fat, Wisecrackers, Roasted Garlic and Rosemary
Partners, A Tasteful Choice Company
800-632-7477 www.partnerscrackers.com
Bottom Line: 110 calories per serving (10 crackers)
Details: Yummy Hunters can't say enough about this discovery. They rave it's the most interesting and delicious cracker they have ever eaten! *Helen:* Oh my God, these are fabulous! *Eric:* So many crackers, so little time before you have to start sharing them.
Availability: Supermarkets and by phone

* Rye
Old London, Melba Snacks, Rye
Old London Foods, Inc.
718-409-1776 www.oldlondonmelba.com
Bottom Line: 60 calories per serving (5 crackers)
Details: Yummy Hunters praise this brand and say they've been eating these crackers forever. They add these crackers have helped them through every diet and say they especially like these Melba Snacks with light cream cheese. *Helen & Eric:* They go great with everything. We tried them with Brummel & Brown strawberry spread and then some melted Polly-O mozzarella. Yum, yum!
Availability: Supermarkets and ordering online at www.efoodpantry.com and www.leesmarket.com

✱ Sesame
Aunt Gussie's, Cracker Flats, Sesame
Aunt Gussie's Cookies and Crackers
800-4-A-Cookie www.auntgussies.com
Bottom Line: 50 calories per serving (1 cracker)
Details: Yummy Hunters say when dieting they get into food ruts. They add these crackers add an exciting and delicious crunch to their otherwise mundane lunch. *Helen & Eric:* We love them plain so we can savor their unique and delicious taste.
Availability: Health food stores and online

✱ Sesame Ginger
Back to Nature, Sesame Ginger, Rice Thins
Back to Nature
866-536-6946 www.backtonaturefoods.com
Bottom Line: 120 calories per serving (29 g)
Details: Yummy Hunters say the subtle flavor of ginger adds a unique taste. *Helen & Eric:* Another ethnic product that adds zest and variety.
Availability: Health food stores and Whole Foods

✱ Whole Grains
Galilee Splendor, Bible Bread, Five Whole Grains
Galilee Splendor
800-819-1223 www.galileesplendor.com
Bottom Line: 120 calories per serving (29 g)
Details: Yummy Hunters rave about the unusual flavor in these whole grain crackers. *Helen:* Full of wheaty freshness. *Eric:* Praise be the Lord!
Availability: Health food stores and Whole Foods

✱ Whole Wheat, Original
Nabisco, Triscuit, Thin Crisps, Original Whole Wheat
Kraft Foods, Inc.
800-622-4726 www.nabiscoworld.com
Bottom Line: 130 calories per serving (15 crackers)
Details: Yummy Hunters love to eat this light, wheaty and crunchy cracker right out of the box. *Helen:* One of my household staples. So light, so crunchy, so good. *Eric:* So, what else did you expect from a Triscuit?
Availability: Supermarkets

RICE CAKES

Corn, Sesame
Real Foods, Organic Corn Thins, Sesame
Real Foods, PTY, LTD
www.cornthins.com
Bottom Line: 45 calories per serving (2 crackers)
Details: Yummy Hunters say it's a great cracker any time of the day. They like it with cream cheese in the AM, tuna salad at lunch and with a dip at dinner. *Helen:* We put a piece of turkey between two crackers and had ourselves a crunchy, low-calorie sandwich. *Eric:* The unique taste and consistency make it very appealing.
Availability: Scattered on the East and West Coasts and online at www.leesmarket.com

* Cracker Jacks
Quaker, Cracker Jacks, Popped Corn Cakes
The Quaker Oats Company
800-856-5781 www.quakeroats.com
Bottom Line: 60 calories per serving (1 cake)
Details: Yummy Hunters ask, Who doesn't remember Cracker Jacks? Another says, every dieter needs an after-dinner treat and this is a favorite. *Helen:* What a find! I'm back in my childhood, too! *Eric:* I ate three and I still can't find the prize!
Availability: Supermarkets

A diet is the penalty we pay for exceeding the feeding limit.

* A Low-Fat Product

CREAMERS

Flavored coffees and teas are all the rage, and our Yummy Hunters have favored us with some flavors that will add zing to your brew. Whether you like the traditional taste of cream or the exoticness of a coffeehouse flavor, we can put cream in anyone's coffee or tea.

---

* Café Mocha
Nestlé, Coffee-Mate, Fat Free, Café Mocha
Nestlé USA, Inc.
800-637-8538 www.coffee-mate.com
Bottom Line: 25 calories per serving (1 tbsp)
Details: Yummy Hunters love the chocolate flavor it gives their coffee. They also love the fact it doesn't add any fat. *Helen & Eric:* It's getting the richness of hot chocolate combined with the jolt of your favorite coffee beans.
Availability: Supermarkets

* Cream
Nature's First, Natural Dairy Creamer
Nature's First, Inc.
800-523-3752 www.naturesfirst.com
Bottom Line: 7 calories per serving (1 packet)
Details: Yummy Hunters brag that they always keep a few creamers with them so when they're in Starbucks they get their coffee black and just pour in the creamer. *Helen:* Really tastes like cream and you can't beat the convenience of this tasty product. *Eric:* Nature or nurture? With this miracle of modern science you don't have to choose.
Availability: Online

✳ Creamer, Non-Dairy
Morningstar Foods, Farm Rich, Fat Free, Non-Dairy Creamer
Dean Foods, Inc.
800-441-3321 www.deanfoods.com
Bottom Line: 10 calories per serving (1 tbsp)
Details: Yummy Hunters tell us it's rich, it's creamy and great for coffee or tea. *Helen & Eric:* Great taste and proves a little can go a long way.
Availability: Supermarkets

✳ Creamora
Bordens, Creamora, Fat Free, Non Dairy Creamer
Dean Foods, Inc.
800-236-1119 www.deanspecialtyfoods.com
Bottom Line: 10 calories per serving (1 tsp)
Details: Yummy Hunters say this product provides unparalleled convenience. They add it makes their coffee creamy and delicious. *Helen:* It gave my coffee a real candy flavor. *Eric:* Creamora, I adore you, me amora.
Availability: Supermarkets

✳ Creamy Chocolate
Nestlé, Coffee-Mate, Fat Free, Creamy Chocolate
Nestlé USA, Inc.
800-637-8538 www.coffee-mate.com
Bottom Line: 50 calories per serving (4 tsp)
Details: Yummy Hunters would rather starve then give up their chocolate fix. *Helen:* I'm a chocoholic. This is the perfect morning mate for my coffee. *Eric:* So that's why you said there wasn't any left.
Availability: Supermarkets

✳ Creme Brulee
Nestlé, Coffee-Mate, Special Edition, Creme Brulee
Nestlé USA, Inc.
800-637-8538 www.coffee-mate.com
Bottom Line: 40 calories per serving (1 tbsp)
Details: Yummy Hunters say one tablespoon gives their coffee a rich, coffeehouse flavor. They also like the toffee nut flavor. *Helen & Eric:* Rich, creamy and oh so heavenly.

Availability: Supermarkets

✳ French Vanilla
International Delight, Fat Free, French Vanilla
Dean Foods, Inc.
800-441-3321 www.internationaldelight.com
Bottom Line: 30 calories per serving (1 tbsp)
Details: Yummy Hunters say they love it because it gives their coffee an exotic, coffeehouse flavor. *Helen:* We love the intense, vanilla aroma. *Eric:* This great creamer knows no boundaries.
Availability: Supermarkets

✳ Half & Half
Land O Lakes, Gourmet, Fat Free, Half & Half
HP Hood, Inc.
800-878-9762 www.landolakes.com
Bottom Line: 20 calories per serving (2 tbsp)
Details: Yummy Hunters confess they used to use skim milk in their coffee to save calories, but when they discovered this product, it gave them a new lease on life. Now they get the real taste of cream without the fat. *Helen:* I had a similar experience; however, to give it a true taste test I prepared two cups of coffee for Eric. One had skim milk, the other Fat Free Half & Half. *Eric:* Nothing halfway about the results — Half & Half, hands down!
Availability: Supermarkets

If it weren't for the fact that the TV set and the refrigerator are so far apart, I wouldn't get any exercise at all.

DIPS

Just as a dip in the water refreshes, the right dip will refresh your foods and your taste buds.

---

* Bean Dip
Bearitos, Fat Free Vegetarian Bean Dip
Hain Celestial Group, Inc.
800-434-4246 www.littlebearfoods.com
Bottom Line: 25 calories per serving (2 tbsp)
Details: Yummy Hunters tell us they are always looking for tasty dips to serve company, so when they discovered this product it became an instant hit. They say it's great with baked tortilla chips.
Helen: I broke out a bag of carrots on this baby!
Eric: South-of-the-border taste, makes me want to break into the Mexican Hat Dance.
Availability: Supermarkets and health food stores

* Chocolate
Walden Farms, Calorie Free, Chocolate Dip
Walden Farms, Inc.
800-229-1706 www.waldenfarms.com
Bottom Line: 0 calories per serving (2 tbsp)
Details: Our Yummy Hunters think it's beyond terrific. They put it on low-fat pancakes and for dessert they mic it, then put it on low-fat ice cream. *Helen & Eric:* We heated it up in the microwave, dipped in some pretzels and they were delicious.
Availability: Supermarkets, health food stores and online

✳ Garlic Herb
Fantastic, Soup & Dip, Recipe Mix, Garlic Herb
Fantastic Foods, Inc.
800-288-1089 www.fantasticfoods.com
Bottom Line: 20 calories per serving (1 cup prepared)
Details: Yummy Hunters recommend mixing
this dip with fat-free sour cream and then eating it
with baked potato chips. One suggests sprinkling a
little on a chicken cutlet before you bake it. *Helen
& Eric:* We made soup using half the amount of
water and tons of fresh veggies. Marvelous!
Availability: Supermarkets, health food stores and
club stores; store locations and ordering online

✳ Marshmallow
Walden Farms, Calorie Free, Marshmallow Dip
Walden Farms, Inc.
800-229-1706 www.waldenfarms.com
Bottom Line: 0 calories per serving (2 tbsp)
Details: A Yummy Hunter tells us she and her sister
used to eat Fluffernutters as kids. Now they're on
a low-carb diet together. When she found this
product, she mixed it with chunky peanut butter,
put it on low-carb bread and she and her sister
were again giggling like little girls. *Helen:* I
remember Fluffernutters, too. Eric had no idea
what they were, so I decided we would make them
as well. *Eric:* OK, I had a deprived childhood.
Anyway, I love 'em.
Availability: Supermarkets, health food stores and
online

✳ Mexican Red Bean
Salpica, Mexican Red Bean Dip
Distributed Frontera Foods, Inc.
800-559-4441 www.fronterakitchens.com
Bottom Line: 15 calories per serving (2 tbsp)
Details: Yummy Hunters say it's the perfect food
to heat up a party. *Helen & Eric:* Just make sure you
have the right low-cal chips if you want your
weight to dip the next day.
Availability: Supermarkets and health food stores;
store locations and ordering online

✳ Nacho Cheese
Mrs. Renfro's, Nacho Cheese Sauce
Renfro's Foods, Inc.
800-332-2456 www.renfrofoods.com
Bottom Line: 30 calories per serving (2 tbsp)
Details: Yummy Hunters pour it over whole wheat pasta and say it makes the most delicious mac and cheese. *Helen & Eric:* Just mic it and dip. We dipped chips, pretzels and veggies and had a blast.
Availability: Supermarkets, gourmet food shops and online

✳ Onion
Walden Farms, Calorie Free, French Onion Dip
Walden Farms, Inc.
800-229-1706 www.waldenfarms.com
Bottom Line: 0 calories per serving (2 tbsp)
Details: Yummy Hunters who love potato chips and onion dip know this combo can be lethal. They're thrilled this dip lets them eat this combo without destroying their diet. *Helen & Eric:* Why stop with chips when you can add your favorite veggies?
Availability: Supermarkets, health food stores and online

✳ Red Pepper
Victoria, Red Pepper Dip
Victoria Packing Corp.
718-927-3000 www.victoriapacking.com
Bottom Line: 50 calories per serving (¼ cup)
Details: Yummy Hunters think these red peppers bring variety to their dipping desires. One says it's been great for her diet. She opens a bag of chips, measures out her portion and dips away. It's one of the ways she managed to lose and maintains a 27-pound weight loss. *Helen & Eric:* Kudos! We love to hear stories like this. This dip rocks.
Availability: Supermarkets and ordering online at www.newyorkflavors.com

Rich, fatty foods are like destiny . . . they, too, shape our ends.

EGGS

Eggs are a magical food and for dieters an elixir of great-tasting meals. Take two simple egg whites, add tomatoes, maybe a little broccoli, light cheese and voila!

---

* Bacon, Egg & Cheese
LEAN POCKETS, Pastries for Breakfast, Bacon, Egg & Cheese
Nestlé USA, Inc.
800-350-5016 www.leanpockets.com
Bottom Line: 150 calories per serving (1 pastry)
Details: Yummy Hunters claim their entire families love these pastries. Yummy Hunters make sure they eat only one; otherwise, they are done for the day. *Eric:* Helen doesn't eat meat, so I had to eat the entire meal by myself. Don't cry for me, Argentina! Do scientists stay up all night to come up with these ingeniously delicious products, or does a lightning bolt just hit them when they're driving on the freeway?
Availability: Supermarkets

Cheese, Egg & Bacon
Pillsbury, Toaster Scrambles, Cheese, Egg & Bacon
General Mills, Inc.
800-828-3291 www.pillsbury.com
Bottom Line: 180 calories per serving (1 pastry)
Details: One overwhelmed new mother told us she only could eat her meals one-handed, so she was overjoyed that this combo solved that problem and also helped her to get her weight down. *Eric:* Another no-no product for Helen and another YES - YES meal for me.
Availability: Supermarkets

✳ Egg & Cheese
Health Is Wealth, Breakfast Munchees, Egg White & Cheese
Val Vasilef, Health Is Wealth Products, Inc.
856-728-1998 www.healthiswealthfoods.com
Bottom Line: 70 calories per serving (2 Munchees)
Details: One Yummy Hunter says every morning she eats four of them on her way to work. She adds it's like eating egg and cheese on a whole wheat roll. *Helen:* Scrambled eggs and cheese wrapped in hot bread. Delicious! *Eric:* If you give me a day or two, I might be able to come up with something.
Availability: Supermarkets and health food stores

✳ Egg & Cheese
Morningstar Farms, Egg & Cheese
Kellogg Co.
800-557-6525 www.morningstarfarms.com
Bottom Line: 280 calories per serving (1 sandwich)
Details: Yummy Hunters say their families will accept no other. *Helen:* Always great to hear how these products satisfy the entire family. *Eric:* So convenient I can yam these down all day.
Availability: Supermarkets

Eggs, Cheddar & Monterey Jack Cheeses
Jimmy Dean, Omelets
Sara Lee Foods
800-925-DEAN www.jimmydean.com
Bottom Line: 210 calories per serving (1 Omelet)
Details: Yummy Hunters say these are great when they're on the go. Others add, high in protein, big on taste. *Helen:* Better than mine for one simple reason, I don't have to clean any pans! *Eric:* A must-try for anyone who loves to make quick and easy omelettes.
Availability: Supermarkets

✳ Egg Whites
Egg Beaters, Egg Whites
ConAgra Foods, Inc.
800-988-7808 www.eggbeaters.com
Bottom Line: 25 calories per serving (3 tbsp)

Details: Yummy Hunters who prepare lots of eggs for their families love this product because now they don't have to separate the egg whites. Others add it removes the temptation to eat the yoke. *Helen:* We made ourselves a Cracker Barrel cheddar omelette — delish. *Eric:* Another ingenious product.
Availability: Supermarkets

✱ Garden Vegetable
Egg Beaters, Garden Vegetable
ConAgra Foods, Inc.
800-988-7808 www.eggbeaters.com
Bottom Line: 30 calories per serving (¼ cup)
Details: Yummy Hunters say they can't tell the difference between this and the real deal. It's so easy, they just open the container and pour! They add they love the garden veggies, which makes for a great omelette. *Helen:* If you're not an egg white person and like that whole-egg taste, I highly encourage you to try this delicious product. *Eric:* I still can't get over the fact eggs come in liquid containers.
Availability: Supermarkets

✱ Sausage, Egg & Cheese
LEAN POCKETS, Pastries for Breakfast, Sausage, Egg & Cheese
Nestlé USA, Inc.
800-350-5016 www.leanpockets.com
Bottom Line: 140 calories per serving (1 pastry)
Details: Yummy Hunters say they get all their favorite ingredients in one low-calorie, take-along breakfast. They add they make it in the toaster oven and eat it in the car on the way to work. *Eric:* The crust cooks up crunchy. I told Helen I'd pick out the sausage, but she told me to keep quiet or she'd pick out another partner.
Availability: Supermarkets

I'm not afraid of heights, I'm afraid of widths.

FISH & SEAFOOD

Fɪsʜ ɪs ʀᴇᴀʟʟʏ ᴛᴇʀʀɪғɪᴄ for dieters. Unfortunately, too many people have a real or imaginary aversion to this food. Our Yummy Hunters have discovered some delicious products and tantalizing ways to integrate fish into anybody's diet regime.

✳ Clams
Bumble Bee, Fancy Whole Baby Clams
Bumble Bee Seafoods, LLC
800-800-8572 www.bumblebee.com
Bottom Line: 50 calories per serving (¼ cup)
Details: Yummy Hunters tell us they love pasta and clam sauce, so they cook some whole wheat pasta, add the clams, a little garlic and very little olive oil and have a wonderfully satisfying meal. *Helen & Eric:* Plump, tasty clams that make a perfect accent to your favorite vegetables and pasta.
Availability: Supermarkets

✳ Crabmeat
Bumble Bee, Premium Select Fancy Lump Crabmeat
Bumble Bee Seafoods, LLC
800-800-8572 www.bumblebee.com
Bottom Line: 40 calories per serving (¼ cup)
Details: Yummy Hunters say they have tried lots of canned crabmeat and it's usually very salty. This one, they say, is perfect and they eat it on crackers or in a salad with a little light mayo. *Helen:* We put it on a bed of lettuce with some Catalina fat-free dressing and we gobbled it down. *Eric:* You can't crab about this crabmeat.
Availability: Supermarkets

* Fish
Dr. Praeger's, Fish Fillets
Ungar's Food Products
201-703-1300 www.drpraegers.com
Bottom Line: 113 calories per serving (1 fillet)
Details: Yummy Hunters say not only is it delicious and low in calories, but it's also kosher. They put it between a light bun with a piece of light cheese and they feel it's their own version of a fast-food meal. *Helen:* It cooked up light and crunchy to make a fresh-tasting meal. *Eric:* Nothing fishy about this delicious dish.
Availability: Supermarkets in 22 states; store locations online and ordering at www.hillersmarket.com

Herring
Brunswick, Boneless Herring Fillets, Seafood Snacks, Kippered
Connors Brunswick
www.brunswick.ca
Bottom Line: 160 calories per serving (1 can)
Details: One Yummy Hunter told us she grew up in Canada and eating these delicious fillets was always a treat. Now that she's living in the States, eating familiar foods helps her stay on her diet. *Helen & Eric:* We put them on Devonshire Mini Bagel Snacks and it made for a tasty snack.
Availability: Supermarkets

Hickory Smoked Tuna
Starkist, Tuna Creations, Hickory Smoked
Starkist Seafood Company
800-252-1587 www.starkist.com
Bottom Line: 80 calories per serving (¼ cup)
Details: Yummy Hunters recommend the smoky flavor and say their families love this new "tuna creation." They add it gives a lift to their tuna salad sandwiches. *Helen:* I've had smoked salmon before, but Hickory Smoked Tuna! What a great new product idea. It really caught our attention. *Eric:* Reel this baby in!
Availability: Supermarkets

Mussels, Smoked
Haddon House, Smoked Mussels
Haddon House Food Products, Inc.
800-257-6174 ext. 225 www.haddonhouse.com
Bottom Line: 95 calories per serving (⅓ cup)
Details: One Yummy Hunter says that when she's dieting this gourmet treat is great on a sandwich with some lettuce and tomato. *Helen:* Terrific woodsy flavor makes these mussels a must-try. FYI, you can cut more calories without cutting the flavor by pouring off some of the oil. *Eric:* I like them with tabasco sauce and a little lemon. When it comes to taste, these little guys have plenty of muscle.
Availability: Gourmet stores

Oysters
3 Diamonds, Whole Oysters
Mitsubishi International Corporation
P.O. Box 800037, San Diego, CA 92138-0037
Bottom Line: 80 calories per serving (2 oz)
Details: One Yummy Hunter raves about how these oysters are so plump and juicy. Others can't believe how fresh they taste and also love how low-cal and filling they are. *Helen:* Restaurant quality. All you need is a little cocktail sauce and you're good to go. I recommend serving them well-chilled. *Eric:* Tender, juicy and full of flavor. Bring on the tartar sauce and some horseradish!
Availability: Supermarkets

Ranch
Gorton's, Ranch Breaded Fish Fillets
Gorton's
800-222-6846 www.gortons.com
Bottom Line: 240 calories per serving (2 fillets)
Details: Yummy Hunters say this gourmet-tasting fish fillet adds excitement to their diet plans. *Helen:* Traditional ranch dressing gives this fish fillet real personality. *Eric:* Try it! This dish will make a fish lover out of almost anybody. The catch of the day!
Availability: Supermarkets

✳ Salmon
Chicken of the Sea, Pink Salmon
Chicken of the Sea, International
www.chickenofthesea.com
Bottom Line: 60 calories per serving (¼ cup)
Details: Yummy Hunters are amazed at the great taste and freshness of this discovery. They tell us they love this salmon over a bed of romaine lettuce with some honey mustard dressing. *Helen:* Fresh, flaky and light tasting. You can open a can and put it on steamed spinach with some mustard sauce or use it to liven up a tossed salad. *Eric:* No matter where you put this delicious salmon, you'll be in the pink!
Availability: Supermarkets, online and ordering at www.netgrocer.com

✳ Salmon
Stouffer's, Lean Cuisine, Spa Cuisine Classics, Salmon with Basil
Nestlé USA, Inc.
800-225-1180 www.leancuisine.com
Bottom Line: 260 calories per serving (9⅝-oz meal)
Details: Salmon-loving Yummy Hunters are overjoyed to finally find a salmon meal that is easy to make and tastes great. *Helen:* This low-fat meal makes for five-star dining in your very own kitchen. *Eric:* Worth opening a bottle of good white wine for this one.
Availability: Supermarkets; store locations online

✳ Salmon, Smoked
Echo Falls Traditional Smoked Salmon
Ocean Beauty Seafoods
973-491-9696 www.oceanbeauty.com
Bottom Line: 100 calories per serving (2 oz)
Details: Yummy Hunters say, not too salty but very tasty and filling. Great for Sunday brunch. *Helen:* All you need are the bagels and low-fat cream cheese. *Eric:* And maybe some tomatoes and onions. Yum, yum!
Availability: Supermarkets and health food stores

Sardines, Lemon
Marco Polo, Sardines with Lemon
Adria Imports, Inc.
718-326-4610   www.adriaimports.com
Bottom Line: 320 calories per serving (4-oz can)
Details: Yummy Hunters who love sardines love the refreshing lemon flavor. One Yummy Hunter says the lemon flavor cuts down the fishiness. *Helen:* The soybean oil and lemon flavor shine through. I drain all the liquid out because that's where the calories swim. *Eric:* We do not want to swim with the calories.
Availability: Online at www.greatfoodz.com

Sardines, Tomato Sauce
Marco Polo, Sardines, Tomato Sauce
Adria Imports, Inc.
718-326-4610   www.adriaimports.com
Bottom Line: 180 calories per serving (4.5 oz)
Details: Yummy Hunters who have been combining sardines and stewed tomatoes finally have their combo in a more convenient can. They rave it's as good as their creations. Yummy Hunters recommend trying some on whole wheat toast with sliced onions. *Helen:* The sweet taste of the tomatoes really enhances the flavor of the sardines. *Eric:* Great sardines, no bones about it.
Availability: Online at www.greatfoodz.com

* Shrimp
Bumble Bee, Premium Select, Deveined Medium Shrimp
Bumble Bee Seafoods, LLC
800-800-8572   www.bumblebee.com
Bottom Line: 40 calories per serving (¼ cup)
Details: Yummy Hunters declare that when dieting they need to pack their own lunch for the office, and this is the perfect alternative to tuna salad. *Helen:* One of the keys to dieting successfully is to plan ahead. These tender, tasty shrimps mixed with light mayo make a fabulous shrimp salad. *Eric:* Perfect size, perfect taste.
Availability: Supermarkets

* Shrimp, Fried Rice
Gorton's, Shrimp Bowl, Fried Rice
Gorton's
800-222-6846 www.gortons.com
Bottom Line: 320 calories per serving (10½ oz)
Details: Yummy Hunters who love fried rice declare this is their favorite lunch. They add that the shrimp are big enough not to get lost in the rice. *Helen:* But wait, I'm eating fried rice! I'm never allowed to eat fried rice on my diet. An incredible find! It tastes like the fried rice I remember eating at my local Chinese restaurant as a kid. *Eric:* When you wish upon a rice bowl . . .
Availability: Supermarkets

* Shrimp, Stir-Fry
Contessa, Shrimp Stir-Fry
Contessa Food Products
888-832-8000 www.contessa.com
Bottom Line: 140 calories per serving (8 oz)
Details: Yummy Hunters say after a hard day at work, this meal is a blessing; it takes just 10 minutes from freezer to dinner table. The family has a delicious hot meal and Yummy Hunters stay on their diet. *Helen:* We ate the entire bag, which added up to 210 calories each. If you're really hungry, this is a great meal. *Eric:* Stir it up.
Availability: Supermarkets; store locations online

Shrimp & Angel Hair Pasta
Stouffer's, Cafe Classics, Shrimp & Angel Hair Pasta
Nestlé USA, Inc.
800-225-1180 www.leancuisine.com
Bottom Line: 240 calories per serving (283 g)
Details: Yummy Hunters say they are reeling with delight now they can have a rich-tasting shrimp and pasta dish without going off their diet plan. *Helen:* Delicate pasta topped with nice-sized and very tasty shrimp. *Eric:* Soft, tender and juicy shrimps in a tasty sauce. Worth a great bottle of white wine.
Availability: Supermarkets; store locations online

✳ Whitefish
Mothers, Whitefish
Rokeach Food Distributors, Inc.
973-491-9696 www.rokeach.com
Bottom Line: 60 calories per serving (1 piece)
Details: Yummy Hunters rave this is the best gefilte fish they have ever had. They serve it to their families on holidays. They add that because they're on a diet, they enjoy it year-round. *Helen:* This traditional Jewish fish appetizer has rocked the diet world. *Eric:* Their recipe is as good as any homemade gefilte fish.
Availability: Kosher section of supermarkets, kosher stores and ordering online at www.netgrocer.com

I'm on a seafood diet. I see food and eat it!

FRUIT

Although we all enjoy fresh fruit, our Yummy Hunters tantalize us with a delicious selection of fruit-based, low-cal products that add the right amount of variety to our diet.

Apple
Crispy Original Apple Chips
Good Health Natural Food, Inc.
631-261-5608 www.e-goodhealth.com
Bottom Line: 140 calories per serving (28 g or 12 chips)
Details: Yummy Hunters say it's a dried fruit that crunches like a chip. They love its originality as much as they love the taste. *Helen:* We think they're better than potato chips. *Eric:* So, shoot us!
Availability: Supermarkets, health food stores and online

* Banana
Nothing But... Banana!
Nothing But... Fruit!
516-629-6433 www.nothingbutfruit.com
Bottom Line: 100 calories per serving (1 oz)
Details: Yummy Hunters say they use these bananas on cereal, in yogurt or right out of the bag. They tell us they have a hard time getting them away from their kids. *Helen:* The sweet taste of banana in a potato chip—like crunch. *Eric:* Another scientific breakthrough! Also comes in pineapple for those who want a taste of Hawaii.
Availability: Online

✳ Fruit Snacks
Planet Harmony, Organic, Fruit Snacks
Harmony Foods Corporation
800-837-2855 www.harmonyfoods.com
Bottom Line: 130 calories per serving (12 pieces)
Details: Yummy Hunters say they love these
because they are naturally chewy and sweet. They
add these snacks fulfill their need to chew when
they're on a diet. *Helen:* Better than any gummy
bear I've ever had! *Eric:* Yep, just like a gummy
bear, but also I remember another similarly
delicious product called Ju Ju Fruits. Chewy, chewy
and chewier.
Availability: Health food stores

✳ Fuji Apple
Crispy Delites, 100% Natural Fruit Chips, Fuji Apple
Healthy Delite
516-593-5369 www.healthydelite.com
Bottom Line: 105 calories per serving (1.07 oz)
Details: *Helen:* Once a Yummy Hunter turned me
onto the celery-flavored veggie chips, I had to
hunt up other products from this company and, lo
and behold, I found this. Sweet, crunchy and fat
free! What more could you ask for? *Eric:* These
guys are geniuses!
Availability: Health food stores and by phone

✳ Mandarin Orange
Del Monte, Mandarin Orange Segments, in Light Syrup
Del Monte Foods
800-543-3090 www.delmonte.com
Bottom Line: 70 calories per serving (1 cup, 113 g)
Details: Yummy Hunters love the sweet taste and
rave about how easy and convenient it is to take
their fruit snacks with them wherever they go.
Helen: Packed in a tasty, light syrup; we love the
delicate flavor of these petite orange slices. *Eric:*
We put them over cottage cheese and created a
mandarin orange delight. What a sweet way to
start the morning.
Availability: Supermarkets and ordering online at
www.netgrocer.com

* Mango
Just Tomatoes, Just Mango
Just Tomatoes
800-537-1985 www.justtomatoes.com
Bottom Line: 90 calories per serving (1 oz)
Details: Yummy Hunters say the taste of mango satisfies their sweet tooth. One ate the entire tub and delighted in the fact it was only 180 calories. *Helen & Eric:* Mango madness!
Availability: Supermarkets, health food stores and online

* Mixed Berrys
Nabisco, 100 Calorie Packs, Fruit Snacks, Mixed Berry
Kraft Foods, Inc.
800-622-4726 www.kraftfoods.com
Bottom Line: 100 calories per serving (1 pckg)
Details: Yummy Hunters confess that on the checkout line they tell the cashier these snacks are for their kids, only they don't have any chilldren. *Helen:* I can see why. Berry, berry sweet but high in sugar! Not a snack for everyday dieters. *Eric:* We take no responsibility for what our Yummy Hunters say or do when they're in a supermarket.
Availability: Supermarkets

* Orange Mango
Musselman's, Lite, No Sugar Added, Orange Mango, Fruit'N Sauce
Knouse Foods, Inc.
717-677-8181 www.knouse.com
Bottom Line: 60 calories per serving (4-oz cup)
Details: Yummy Hunters are delirious over this gourmet fruit blend. *Helen:* Orange and mangoes give this traditional applesauce a tropical flavor. I like the fact that it relies on the fruit's natural sweetness without adding any sugar. *Eric:* Where was this product when I was growing up? No wonder I felt unhappy and deprived. Orange mango is helping me work through some of these issues.
Availability: Some supermarkets; store locations online

* Peach
Mott's, Healthy Harvest, Peach Medley
Mott's, Inc.
800-426-4891 www.motts.com
Bottom Line: 50 calories per serving (1 cup)
Details: Yummy Hunters declare this is as good as it gets! They add it's refreshingly delicious. *Helen & Eric:* Imagine a cup of applesauce with a natural peachy flavor!
Availability: Supermarkets

* Peaches, Strawberry, Banana
Del Monte, Lite Fruit and Gel, Peaches in Strawberry-Banana Gel
Del Monte Foods
800-543-3090 www.delmonte.com
Bottom Line: 60 calories per serving (1 cup)
Details: Yummy Hunters say this reminds them of the gelatin molds their moms used to make for the neighborhood picnics. Now the roles are reversed and Yummy Hunters serve them to their moms and their own kids. *Helen:* Perfect combo of sweet gelatin and the fresh taste of fruit. I love 'em for breakfast or as an after-dinner treat. *Eric:* Great with cottage cheese or with a little low-fat whipped cream.
Availability: Supermarkets

* Pears
Nothing But... Pears
Nothing But... Fruit!
516-629-6433 www.nothingbutfruit.com
Bottom Line: 70 calories per serving (1 package)
Details: Yummy Hunters who are looking for something sweet and who love the taste of pears say this is their favorite snack. One eats it when travelling. Another adds it's become a favorite in her office. *Helen:* If you're looking for something sweet but without guilt, these crunchy pears do the trick. *Eric:* I can enjoy the taste of pears all year round. Nothing but . . . delicious.
Availability: Online

* Pineapple
Dole, Pineapple Chunks in Pineapple Juice
Dole
www.dole.com
Bottom Line: 60 calories per serving (½ cup)
Details: Yummy Hunters think it's so much easier than cutting up a pineapple. They love to put them in an ice cube tray and freeze them. *Helen:* One bite says it all! Eric likes to drink the juice right out of the jar—what a P.I.G.! *Eric:* Also available in convenient fruit bowls, which are just as easy to drink out of. Oink, oink!
Availability: Supermarkets and ordering online at www.netgrocer.com

* Pineapple
Made In Nature, Pineapple
Made In Nature
559-445-8601 www.madeinature.com
Bottom Line: 130 calories per serving (¼ cup)
Details: Yummy Hunters say these small, bite-sized chunks of fruit taste just like candy. *Helen:* Sure to satisfy anyone's sweet tooth. *Eric:* The more I ate, the more I appreciated the deliciousness of this product.
Availability: Supermarkets and health food stores

* Raspberry
Stretch Island, Fruit Leather, Rare Raspberry
Stretch Island
www.stretch-island.com
Bottom Line: 45 calories per serving (½-oz pckg)
Details: Yummy Hunters love the authentic raspberry taste. They add it's so convenient to keep these treats in their bags or desk drawers. Others say it's a funky snack and great for their kids' lunch boxes. *Helen:* Another fun product. I love to take it to the movies. *Eric:* They know how to "stretch" out the fruity taste. Muncho Mango is another yummy flavor.
Availability: Health food stores, many supermarkets and in some warehouse club stores; online and at www.truefoodsonline.com

✻ Strawberry
Just Tomatoes, Just Strawberries
Just Tomatoes
800-537-1985 www.justtomatoes.com
Bottom Line: 150 calories per serving (1 container)
Details: Yummy Hunters love this brand. They told us about the peach flavor (see previous listing) and this strawberry version, which they consider to be their favorite dried-fruit snack. *Helen & Eric:* We love the way it combines a fun crunch with a fabulous fruit flavor.
Availability: Supermarkets, health food stores and online

✻ Strawberry
Kettle Valley, Fruit Snack, Strawberry
Kettle Valley
888-297-6944 www.kettlevalley.net
Bottom Line: 68 calories per serving (1 snack)
Details: Yummy Hunters declare this is their favorite in-between-meal snack. Others rave it's sweet and delicious and say they have a hard time getting it away from their kids. *Helen:* An apple a day keeps the doctor away, and Kettle Valley says there is an apple in every one of its snacks. *Eric:* Beat the kettle drum because this Kettle comes in seven fabulous flavors.
Availability: Supermarkets on the West Coast, online and ordering at www.givemefood.com

✻ Tropical
Blackbird, Fruit Veggies Crunchies, Tropical
Blackbird Food Co.
805-565-4625 www.blackbirdfood.com
Bottom Line: 98 calories per serving (¾ cup)
Details: Yummy Hunters use this to sweeten up their corn flakes. *Helen:* I love the taste plain. *Eric:* A mixture of delicious flavors in every crunch.
Availability: Online

To lengthen your life, shorten your meals.
—Proverb

GELATIN

JELL-O, PUDDINGS

W HEN YOU NEED to hold your diet together, nothing does the trick better or with more flavor than gelatin. Our Yummy Hunters have discovered some old standbys as well as some innovative new products.

JELL-O

✱ Peaches, Strawberry, Banana
Del Monte, Peaches, Strawberry, Banana Gel
Del Monte Foods
800-543-3090 www.delmonte.com
Bottom Line: 70 calories per serving (1 cup)
Details: Yummy Hunters say this reminds them of the gelatin molds their moms used to make for neighborhood picnics. Now the roles are reversed, and Yummy Hunters serve them to their moms and their own kids. *Helen:* Perfect combo of sweet gelatin and the fresh taste of fruit. I love 'em for breakfast or as an after-dinner treat. *Eric:* Great with cottage cheese or with a little low-fat whipped cream.
Availability: Supermarkets and ordering online at www.netgrocer.com

✱ Raspberry
Jolly Rancher, Sugar Free, Gel Snacks, Raspberry
ConAgra Foods, Inc.
800-957-3339 www.huntssnackpack.com
Bottom Line: 10 calories per serving (1 cup, 92 g)
Details: Yummy Hunters who love Jolly Rancher candies say these taste the same, only they're sugar-free gel. *Helen & Eric:* Tastes like the candy to us. We love it!
Availability: Supermarkets

✱ Strawberry
Jell-O, Sugar Free, Strawberry Gelatin
Kraft Foods, Inc.
800-538-1998 www.kraftfoods.com
Bottom Line: 10 calories per serving (1 box)
Details: Yummy Hunters love the convenience of having Jell-O whenever they want it and say it's the best emergency diet food ever. *Helen:* I hear you; I've had some of those diet emergencies myself. *Eric:* I don't know from diet emergencies, but I do know this wonderful product also comes in other delicious flavors.
Availability: Supermarkets

PUDDINGS

✱ Butterscotch
Jell-O, Sugar Free, Fat Free, Instant Butterscotch
Kraft Foods, Inc.
800-538-1998 www.kraftfoods.com
Bottom Line: 25 calories per serving (¼ pack)
Details: Yummy Hunters love the way this wonderful treat makes up in 5 minutes. It's a terrific last-minute dessert. *Helen:* The taste of butterscotch candy and the creaminess of pudding make this one dessert you won't want to pass up. *Eric:* We loved the butterscotch so much, we tried the other flavors and they were equally as good.
Availability: Supermarkets

✱ Chocolate-Vanilla
Jell-O, Fat Free, Pudding Snacks, Chocolate-Vanilla Swirls
Kraft Foods, Inc.
800-538-1998 www.kraftfoods.com
Bottom Line: 100 calories per serving (1 cup)
Details: Yummy Hunters who diet confess it's hard to choose vanilla over chocolate. Now, they don't have to. *Helen:* If you dip your spoon in right, you'll get the perfect amount of chocolate and vanilla in each spoonful. Two Yums Up! *Eric:* Our next book will be about how to correctly dip your spoon.
Availability: Supermarkets

* Mixed Berries
Jell-O, Smoothie Snacks, Mixed Berries
Kraft Foods, Inc.
800-538-1998   www.kraftfoods.com
Bottom Line: 100 calories per serving (1 cup)
Details: Yummy Hunters who love smoothies can't resist these snacks. One declares she lost 75 pounds and this is helping her to keep it off. *Helen & Eric:* Fruity and deliciously smooth. P.S. Hats off to our Yummy Hunter!
Availability: Supermarkets

* Rice
Kozy Shack, Original, Rice Pudding
Kozy Shack, Inc.
www.kozyshack.com
Bottom Line: 130 calories per serving (1 pudding cup, 113 g)
Details: Yummy Hunters rave this is the best rice pudding they've ever had. They add they don't need to make homemade rice pudding anymore. *Helen:* What a terrific product. Make sure to stay to your portion size—this is dangerously delicious. *Eric:* I like to put a little on my tongue and let it slowly dissolve until I feel I'm being lifted up to pudding heaven. Is there anything wrong with that?
Availability: Supermarkets

* Strawberry and Creme
Jell-O, Crème Savers, Pudding Snacks, Strawberry and Creme
Kraft Foods, Inc.
800-538-1998   www.kraftfoods.com
Bottom Line: 130 calories per serving (1 cup)
Details: Yummy Hunters who love crème saver candies tell us these are every bit as delicious. *Helen & Eric:* And they certainly are! A really savory sweet treat.
Availability: Supermarkets

Brain cells come and brain cells go, but fat cells live forever.

GUM

Every dieter knows you can't chew gum and eat at the same time.

————————————

✳ Berry Bubble
Trident-For Kids, Berry, Bubble Gum
Cadbury Adams, Division of Warner-Lambert Co.
800-524-2854 www.cadburyadams.com
Bottom Line: 5 calories per serving (1 stick)
Details: One Yummy Hunter originally bought it for her seven-year-old daughter after a trip to the dentist, but now she buys an additional pack for herself. They both love the fruity, bubble gum taste. *Helen:* The wonderful aromatic smell gets you the minute you open the package. *Eric:* Juicy, juicy and more juicy.
Availability: Any place gum is sold

✳ Bubble
Bazooka, Sugarless, Bubble Gum
Topps Company
www.topps.com
Bottom Line: 20 calories per serving (1 piece)
Details: Yummy Hunters say when they're dieting cracking gum and blowing bubbles relieves the stress and provides some much-needed fun. *Helen:* I hate to burst Eric's bubble, but mine are bigger. *Eric:* And who's using two pieces? Sweetest bubbles you'll ever blow.
Availability: Any place gum is sold

* Cinnamon
Trident, Sugarless Gum, Cinnamon
Cadbury Adams, Division of Warner-Lambert Co.
800-524-2854 www.cadburyadams.com
Bottom Line: 5 calories per serving (1 stick)
Details: Yummy Hunters rave about the authentic and long-lasting cinnamon flavor. *Helen & Eric:* One of the most common baking spices, cinnamon makes for a deliciously sweet and enduring chewing gum flavor.
Availability: Any place gum is sold

* Citrus Samba
Chiclets, Sugarless Gum, Citrus Samba
Cadbury Adams, Division of Warner-Lambert Co.
800-524-2854 www.cadburyadams.com
Bottom Line: 5 calories per serving (2 pieces)
Details: Yummy Hunters say this is the perfect after-meal sweet. *Helen:* Deliciously mouth watering. *Eric:* Wowee! It's making us dance the samba!
Availability: Any place gum is sold

* Citrus Splash
Carefree, Koolerz, Sugar Free, Citrus Splash
Hershey Foods Corp.
800-468-1714 www.koolerz.com
Bottom Line: 5 calories per serving (1 piece)
Details: Yummy Hunters love the intense flavor and say it's a really amazing experience. *Helen:* It has an orangey and refreshing flavor, different from anything we have ever had. I just discovered the watermelon flavor and I'm in heaven. *Eric:* A splash hit! Also comes in mouth-watering berry.
Availability: Any place gum is sold

* Cool Rush
Trident, Sugarless Gum, Cool Rush
Cadbury Adams, Division of Warner-Lambert Co.
800-524-2854 www.cadburyadams.com
Bottom Line: 5 calories per serving (1 stick)
Details: Yummy Hunters like the refreshing flavor and say chewing gum keeps their mouths busy, and

busy mouths can't eat anything. *Helen:* A rush of delicious flavor in every piece. Chewing gum sure has come a long way from the time early American settlers chewed spruce sap and beeswax. *Eric:* They chewed what?
Availability: Any place gum is sold

* Polarice
Wrigley's, Extra, Sugarfree Gum, Polarice
WM Wrigley Jr., Co.
800-974-4539 www.wrigley.com
Bottom Line: 5 calories per serving (1 stick)
Details: Yummy Hunters rave about the cool, minty flavor that seems to go on forever. One Yummy Hunter who cooks with a lot of garlic keeps this by her side so the minute she steps out of the kitchen she knows her breath is fresh and clean. *Helen:* The minty taste refreshes and cleans my mouth at the same time. *Eric:* Icing on the gum!
Availability: Any place gum is sold

* Spearmint
Trident, White, Sugarless Gum, Spearmint
Cadbury Adams, Division of Warner-Lambert Co.
800-524-2854 www.cadburyadams.com
Bottom Line: 5 calories per serving (2 pieces)
Details: Yummy Hunters who are on low-carb diets tell us they always have a bad taste in their mouths and this gum not only freshens their breath but also whitens their teeth. *Helen & Eric:* Exploding in deliciously juicy spearmint flavor.
Availability: Any place gum is sold

* Wild Berry Frost
Wrigley's, Extra, Sugarfree Gum, Wild Berry Frost
WM Wrigley Jr., Co.
800-974-4539 www.wrigley.com
Bottom Line: 5 calories per serving (1 stick)
Details: Yummy Hunters go wild over this refreshing and unique-tasting gum. *Helen & Eric:* Really interesting and stimulating taste.
Availability: Any place gum is sold

* Wintergreen

Dentyne, Ice, Sugarless Gum, Wintergreen

Cadbury Adams, Division of Warner-Lambert Co.
800-524-2854   www.cadburyadams.com

Bottom Line: 5 calories per serving (2 pieces)

Details: Yummy Hunters love the first chew and the burst of cool ice flavor. *Helen & Eric:* We agree. This is a perky piece of deliciousness.

Availability: Any place gum is sold

I'm on a 90-day wonder diet. Thus far, I've lost 45 days.

HOT DOGS

Hot dog! Our Yummy Hunters have discovered some really delicious products that make us think of baseball and barbecues. These are real "wieners"!

---

* Beef
Hebrew National, 97% Fat Free, Beef Franks
ConAgra Foods, Inc.
800-457-6649 www.hebrewnational.com
Bottom Line: 45 calories per serving (1 frank)
Details: Yummy Hunters say they have always trusted Hebrew National to produce a high-quality great-tasting hot dog and they recommend these light beef franks because they live up to that great standard. *Eric:* I had one on a light bun with Boar's Head mustard and Sabrett's Onion Sauce. The one downer was Helen made sure I took small bites. Man, anyone knows that something so delicious has to be shoved whole into your mouth.
Availability: Supermarkets

* Beef, Pork & Turkey
Ball Park, Fat Free, Franks, Beef, Pork & Turkey
Ballpark Brands
888-317-5867 www.ballparkfranks.com
Bottom Line: 40 calories per serving (1 frank)
Details: Yummy Hunters say these dogs have it all. Low in calories and a great mixture of meats make this a great win. *Eric:* This dog has me singing "Take me out to the ball game."
Availability: Supermarkets

∗ Smoked White Turkey
Ball Park, Fat Free, Smoked White Turkey Franks
Ballpark Brands
888-317-5867 www.ballparkfranks.com
Bottom Line: 45 calories per serving (1 frank)
Details: Yummy Hunters love the smoky, barbecue flavor. *Helen & Eric:* For 45 calories, this is a really special find. We each had two franks with Boar's Head mustard and some Sabrett onions on top. This was amazingly filling and oh-so-tasty!
Availability: Supermarkets

∗ Turkey
Applegate Farms, Natural, Uncured Turkey Hot Dogs
Applegate Farms
866-587-5858 www.applegatefarms.com
Bottom Line: 120 calories per serving (1 hot dog)
Details: For flavor and natural goodness, Yummy Hunters like them better than beef hot dogs. *Helen:* We split them down the middle and then melted fat-free cheese on top. *Eric:* They looked and smelled so good, we held off eating them for a good 10 seconds.
Availability: Health food stores; store locations and ordering online

∗ Turkey and Beef
Oscar Mayer, Fat Free Wieners Made with Turkey and Beef
Oscar Mayer Foods Corp.
800-222-2323 www.oscarmayer.com
Bottom Line: 40 calories per serving (1 link)
Details: Yummy Hunters love these because they're a little sweeter than the normal hot dog. One says she likes volume and loves the fact that she can eat two. *Eric:* Three, do I hear three?
Availability: Supermarkets

∗ Veggie, Corn
Morningstar Farms, Veggie Corn Dogs
Kellogg Co.
800-557-6525 www.morningstarfarms.com
Bottom Line: 170 calories per serving (1 dog)

Details: Yummy Hunters love the taste of these corn dogs. They dip them in spicy brown mustard and tell us not only are they tasty, but they're fun to eat. *Helen:* What a unique product. Deliciously filling and oh-so-fun. *Eric:* This dog's got one delicious pedigree!

Availability: Supermarkets

I'm in shape. Round is a shape . . . isn't it?

ICE CREAM
BOWLS, ICE CREAM, ICES

I<small>T'S THE ULTIMATE</small> red-light food. Linked to our subconscious by the bells of the Ice Cream Truck, it's the à la mode on the pie and what makes a cherry come alive. Our Yummy Hunters got the picture and provided us with a lot of green-light choices.

BOWLS

* Waffle
Keebler Waffle Bowls
Keebler
877-453-5837 www.keebler.com
Bottom Line: 50 calories per serving (1 bowl)
Details: *Helen:* A friend shared these with me and I was hooked. She put in low-fat ice cream, but I went one better and added lite Kool Whip. When I serve them, everyone thinks I'm such a gourmet. *Eric:* When the ice cream's gone, you can feast on the ice-cream-soaked waffle! These are great!
Availability: Supermarkets

ICE CREAM

* Brownie Bliss
Healthy Choice, Premium, Low-Fat Ice Cream, Brownie Bliss
ConAgra Foods, Inc.
800-323-9980 www.healthychoice.com
Bottom Line: 130 calories per serving (½ cup)
Details: Yummy Hunters say every spoonful gives a chocolate sensation. Others add it's creamy and smooth and has melt-in-your-mouth goodness. *Helen:* We can't even go there when we talk portion control on this baby! *Eric:* Keep some dignity as you shovel the spoon in and out of the carton.
Availability: Supermarkets

* Caramel Swirl
Healthy Choice, Premium Caramel Swirl Sandwiches
ConAgra Foods, Inc.
800-323-9980 www.healthychoice.com
Bottom Line: 140 calories per serving (1 sandwich)
Details: Our Yummy Hunters rave and say it is better than any fattening ice cream they have ever had. Some carefully remove the cracker layer and take a couple of licks off the smooth and creamy filling before they replace the tasty top. *Helen:* Premium vanilla ice cream with a sweet caramel swirl. *Eric:* Do our Yummy Hunters know how to eat ice cream, or what? Give this swirl a whirl.
Availability: Supermarkets

* Chocolate Cherry Mambo
Healthy Choice, Chocolate Cherry Mambo, Ice Cream
ConAgra Foods, Inc.
800-323-9980 www.healthychoice.com
Bottom Line: 120 calories per serving (½ cup)
Details: Yummy Hunters say it's like eating chocolate-covered cherries! *Helen:* The taste of chocolate-covered cherries in rich creamy ice cream. Need I say more? *Eric:* We polished off the whole container before we could see anything but the glint from our spoons. Let our shameful behavior be a lesson to you all.
Availability: Supermarkets

* Chocolate Eclair
No Pudge!, Giant Chocolate Eclair
No Pudge!
800-423-2763 www.nopudge.com
Bottom Line: 110 calories per serving (1 bar)
Details: Yummy Hunters say this is reminiscent of a childhood favorite and every bit as good. *Helen:* A delicious crunchy outer layer covers a rich, creamy ice cream center. Yummy! *Eric:* Giant Chocolate Eclair—heart be still! Can you believe this is on anyone's diet plan!
Availability: Supermarkets, health food stores; store locations online

Chocolate Fudge
Weight Watchers, Giant Sundae Cones, Chocolate Fudge
Wells Dairy, Inc.
800-331-0830 www.betterforme.com
Bottom Line: 140 calories per serving (1 cone)
Details: Yummy Hunters declare it's like the ice cream they got from the ice cream truck when they were little. The fact that it's only 2 points on Weight Watchers makes it even more delicious. *Helen & Eric:* We never would have thought in a million years that an ice cream cone could have been on someone's diet. This is unbelievable! They also make this in vanilla.
Availability: Supermarkets

✳ Cookies 'N Cream
The Skinny Cow Bar, Cookies 'N Cream
Dryer's Grand Ice Cream, Inc.
888-442-3722 www.skinnycow.com
Bottom Line: 120 calories per serving (1 bar)
Details: Yummy Hunters say, Thank you, Skinny Cow, for they've become Cookies 'N Cream addicts. They love that this was created for dieters. *Helen:* Delicious Cookies 'N Cream ice cream on a portion-controlled stick. *Eric:* Yeah. That's if you stick to one stick, which I didn't. Help me, please! *Helen:* You ate them, not me. What is, is best.
Availability: Supermarkets

✳ Creamy Coconut
Tropicana, Chunks Of Fruit, Creamy Coconut
Integrated Brands, Inc.
800-423-2763 www.coolbrandsinternational.com
Bottom Line: 110 calories per serving (1 bar)
Details: Yummy Hunters who love frozen fruit pops choose this as their favorite. *Helen:* Frozen creamy coconut on a stick. I love the way it has real chunks of fruit in every bite. *Eric:* You'll have to pick the coconut chunks out of your teeth when you're done with this winner. If an ice cream bar melts in the forest, does anybody get fat?
Availability: Supermarkets

* Fudgy
No Pudge!, Giant Fudgy Bar
No Pudge!
800-423-2763 www.nopudge.com
Bottom Line: 60 calories per serving (1 bar)
Details: Yummy Hunters tell us they first got wind of this delicious 0-point goody at their Weight Watchers meeting. They add it's a smooth chocolate sensation on a stick. *Helen:* Jam-packed with fudgy goodness. *Eric:* I'm thinking of freezing one and seeing how long it takes me to lick myself into a chocolate coma?
Availability: Supermarkets, health food stores; store locations online

Jumpin' Java
Healthy Choice, Jumpin' Java, Ice Cream
ConAgra Foods, Inc.
800-323-9980 www.healthychoice.com
Bottom Line: 130 calories per serving (½ cup)
Details: Yummy Hunters say this reminds them of Baskin-Robbins Jamoca Almond Fudge ice cream. They both are loaded with fudge and nuts, but the Healthy Choice isn't loaded with calories. *Helen:* Beware of portion overload, or your spoon will be jumping nonstop into the java. *Eric:* All I want to know is, when I get to heaven, can I eat all the Jumpin' Java I want without getting fat?
Availability: Supermarkets

* Mocha
Starbucks Coffee, Frappuccino, Mocha, Low Fat, Ice Cream Bars
Starbucks Ice Cream Partnership
800-558-7328 www.starbucksicecream.com
Bottom Line: 120 calories per serving (1 bar)
Details: Yummy Hunters say this is the ultimate frozen coffee pop! *Helen:* Although we love to have a Frappuccino in the afternoon at Starbucks, these bars last longer and taste just as good! *Eric:* And, no lines!
Availability: Supermarkets

* Orange Cream
Tropicana, Real Fruit Orange & Cream Bars
Integrated Brands, Inc.
800-423-2763 www.coolbrandsinternational.com
Bottom Line: 80 calories per serving (1 bar)
Details: Yummy Hunters confess these remind them of the mouth-watering Creamsicle pops they had as kids. *Helen:* Refreshing, sweet orange sherbert covering a creamy, vanilla center. This takes us back to our childhood and memories of carefree hot summer days. *Eric:* Ever try sucking out the vanilla while keeping the outer shell intact? I'm still trying.
Availability: Supermarkets

* Orange/Raspberry
Healthy Choice, Premium Sorbet and Cream Bars, Orange or Raspberry
ConAgra Foods, Inc.
800-323-9980 www.healthychoice.com
Bottom Line: 90 calories per serving (1 bar)
Details: Yummy Hunters say the swirl effect gives them the perfect bite of fruit and cream. *Helen & Eric:* It's rich, creamy and refreshing and once again reminds us of the old-time Creamsicles that were oh-so-delicious.
Availability: Supermarkets

* Strawberry Shortcake
No Pudge!, Giant Strawberry Shortcake
No Pudge!
800-423-2763 www.nopudge.com
Bottom Line: 110 calories per serving (1 bar)
Details: Yummy Hunters jump for joy over this delicious ice cream that is only 2 points on Weight Watchers. *Helen:* A world of swirling strawberries in a crunchy coating. *Eric:* Helen swears I didn't use any utensils and just shoved it in my mouth, but anyone who truly knows the real me would know that is just a bald-faced lie. Excuse me while I wash the strawberry rings off my face.
Availability: Supermarkets and health food stores

✱ Sundae Chocolate Fudge
Weight Watchers, Giant Chocolate Fudge Sundae Cup
Wells Dairy, Inc.
800-331-0830 www.betterforme.com
Bottom Line: 160 calories per serving (1 cup)
Details: Yummy Hunters love this sundae cup with its ample amount of rich chocolate fudge. They add it takes so long to eat, when they're finished they're full for the day. *Helen & Eric:* Big is good! Chocolate is good! Fudge is good! It's all good!
Availability: Supermarkets

✱ Vanilla/Chocolate
Silhouette, Vanilla/Chocolate Ice Cream Sandwich
Dryer's Grand Ice Cream, Inc.
888-442-3722 www.skinnycow.com
Bottom Line: 130 calories per serving (1 sandwich)
Details: Yummy Hunters tell us it reminds them of the flying saucers they ate as a kid. They add that they like to roll the sides in chocolate sprinkles. *Helen:* The ice cream is creamy and the cookie is soft and scrumptious. We bought the combo pack (chocolate and vanilla) and couldn't decide which one we loved more. *Eric:* I like to leave a sandwich out until it almost melts and then just lick it up. I think I'm part cat. Available in other flavors, one more delicious than the next.
Availability: Supermarkets

✱ Vanilla/Chocolate, Vanilla/Strawberry
Silhouette, Ice Cream Sundae Cups
Dryer's Grand Ice Cream, Inc.
888-442-3722 www.skinnycow.com
Bottom Line: 120 calories per serving (1 cup strawberry); 130 calories per serving (1 cup chocolate)
Details: One Yummy Hunter says, "If you watched my family eating desserts, you'd never know we're all on diets." *Helen:* Great little ice cream sundae cups—and I do mean little. One really satisfies me, but if you're looking for a big dessert, you may want two. *Eric:* Diet? These are diet!?!
Availability: Supermarkets

Vanilla with Nestlé Crunch Coating
Nestlé, Crunch Reduced Fat Ice Cream Bars, Vanilla
Nestlé's Ice Cream Co., LLC
800-441-2525 www.nestle-icecream.com
Bottom Line: 150 calories per serving (1 bar)
Details: Yummy Hunters say it's the perfect combination of a Nestlé Crunch Bar and creamy vanilla ice cream. *Helen:* Creamy, crunchy and chocolatey—everything we love in a pop! *Eric:* It's a Nestlé Crunch Bar with vanilla ice cream! My God, the idea is enough to drive you crazy! Give these guys a "Nobel Food Prize."
Availability: Supermarkets

ICES

✴ Grape and Cherry
Cool Fruits, Fruit Juice Freezers, Grape and Cherry
nSpired Natural Foods
510-686-0116 www.nspiredfoods.com
Bottom Line: 70 calories per serving (3 pops)
Details: Yummy Hunters like the fact that their kids love this fruit-based product. They confess they eat them, too. One Yummy Hunter recently quit smoking and found these a perfect nighttime replacement that didn't cause a weight gain. *Helen & Eric:* Not only is it all natural, it tastes delicious as well. Kudos to our Yummy Hunter who stopped smoking! We know how hard that is!
Availability: Online at www.givemefood.com

✴ Lemon
Froz Fruit, Gourmet Frozen Fruit Bar, Lemon
Froz Fruit Company
888-700-4700 www.frozfruit.com
Bottom Line: 80 calories per serving (1 bar)
Details: Yummy Hunters tell us it's so, so refreshing. One says it's a good palate cleanser. *Helen:* It's like Grandma's lemonade. *Eric:* Great choice on a hot summer's day.
Availability: Supermarkets, delis and Hershey's ice cream parlors

✳ Orange, Cherry and Grape
Sugar Free, Popsicle, Orange, Cherry and Grape
Good Humor-Breyers
888-707-8737 www.popsicle.com
Bottom Line: 15 calories per serving (1 pop)
Details: Yummy Hunters tell us nothing cools them down on a hot day better than ices. They like to eat one of each flavor, for 45 calories! *Helen:* Great fruity flavor and deliciously refreshing. *Eric:* Their website has a lot of great games, too! (When you play games, you don't eat!)
Availability: Supermarkets

✳ Strawberry
Dr. Praeger's, Sensible Treats Strawberry Pop
Ungar's Food Products
201-703-1300 www.drpraegers.com
Bottom Line: 60 calories per serving (1 pop)
Details: Yummy Hunters who love ices say this is one sweet treat. *Helen:* It's like eating a frozen strawberry. *Eric:* I like to take a bite, crunch it around in my mouth and then slurp it down. Of course, I like to do this when I'm alone.
Availability: Supermarkets in 22 states; store locations online and ordering at www.hillersmarket.com

✳ Strawberry
Froz Fruit Gourmet Frozen Fruit Bar, Chunky Strawberry
Froz Fruit Company
888-700-4700 www.frozfruit.com
Bottom Line: 90 calories per serving (1 bar)
Details: Yummy Hunters rave about great ices and say the name tells it all! *Helen:* Delicious, real chunks of strawberry make it superdelicious. *Eric:* We like having strawberries in season, all year long.
Availability: Supermarkets, delis and Hershey's ice cream parlors (located in 23 states)

Stressed spelled backward is ***desserts***. Coincidence? I think not!

LUNCH MEATS

Lunch meats or colds cuts — no matter what you call them or how you slice them, they are something we grew up with and as dieters want to keep enjoying. So, enjoy!

* Black Forest Smoked Ham
Tyson, Self-Serve Deli Meats, Black Forest Smoked Ham
Tyson Foods, Inc.
800-233-6332 www.tyson.com
Bottom Line: 30 calories per serving (1 slice)
Details: Yummy Hunters ham it up over this product, saying it has mouth-watering flavor.
Eric: Tender and juicy. I agree, ham it up.
Availability: Supermarkets

* Corn Beef
Tyson, Self-Serve Deli Meats, Corn Beef
Tyson Foods, Inc.
800-233-6332 www.tyson.com
Bottom Line: 70 calories per serving (2 slices)
Details: Yummy Hunters say it makes a very hearty sandwich when put between two pieces of rye with some lettuce and mustard. *Eric:* If you love corn beef, this deli delight is for you.
Availability: Supermarkets

✱ Honey Ham
Healthy Choice, Deluxe Thin Sliced, Honey Ham
ConAgra Foods, Inc.
800-323-9980 www.healthychoice.com
Bottom Line: 60 calories per serving (7 slices)
Details: Yummy Hunters love the superthin slices that are so full of taste. Another just likes the fact that now she can eat a ham sandwich and still be on her diet. *Eric:* I made a honey of a wrap with ham, fat-free cheese, mustard on one side and light mayo on the other. Poor Helen, she doesn't know what she's missing.
Availability: Supermarkets

✱ Honey Roasted & Smoked Turkey
Tyson, Self-Serve Deli Meats, Honey Roasted & Smoked Turkey Breast
ConAgra Foods, Inc.
800-457-6649 www.healthychoice.com
Bottom Line: 60 calories per serving (4 slices)
Details: Yummy Hunters tell us that the smoked flavor really packs a punch! One adds this turkey to a chopped salad with her own low-fat honey mustard dressing and says it's sensational. *Helen:* Turkey with a sweet, smoky flavor. We tried it on pita bread with a few pickles. It made a smoky, pickle-packin' sandwich. *Eric:* Try to say that 10 times fast.
Availability: Supermarkets

✱ Mesquite Turkey
Healthy Choice, Mesquite Turkey Breast
ConAgra Foods, Inc.
800-457-6649 www.healthychoice.com
Bottom Line: 60 calories per serving (4 slices)
Details: Yummy Hunters say this is a new and exciting way to eat turkey. One puts four slices on a slice of whole wheat bread and melts a piece of low-fat American cheese on top. *Helen:* Mild flavor with a subtle mesquite taste makes for a gourmet lunch meat. *Eric:* Give your lunch a kick with this Wild West sensation.
Availability: Supermarkets

* Peanut, Thai, Meatless Jerky
Primal Strips, Seitan, Thai Peanut
Primal Spirit Foods
800-887-6162 www.primalspiritfoods.com
Bottom Line: 74 calories per serving (1 oz)
Details: Yummy Hunters say this is a high-protein, exotic-tasting, low-calorie snack that really fills them up. *Helen:* Exciting and different. Like nothing I've every had before. *Eric:* Don't be a jerk, this jerky is a real treat.
Availability: Supermarkets and health food stores

* Roasted Turkey
Applegate, Roasted Turkey Breast
Applegate Farms
866-587-5858 www.applegatefarms.com
Bottom Line: 50 calories per serving (2 oz)
Details: Yummy Hunters say they eat a lot of salads when they're dieting, and these tasty turkey breasts really complement their greens. *Helen:* Fresh turkey that tastes like it was just sliced off the bone. This is a wonderful addition to sandwiches and salads. *Eric:* I rolled a slice and spread some light mayo on it. Then I made another, and another.
Availability: Health food stores; store locations and ordering online

* Smoked Turkey
Hillshire Farm, Deli Select, Thin Sliced, Smoked Turkey Breast
Sara Lee
800-328-2426 www.hillshirefarm.com
Bottom Line: 50 calories per serving (6 slices)
Details: Yummy Hunters who grew up eating cold cuts need their slice meats when dieting, and this smoked turkey breast is a great alternative. *Helen:* It has a lighter smoky taste than some of the others we've tried, but it could be because the slices were very thin. Nevertheless, still very tasty. *Eric:* Thin is good. I wrapped it around a carrot stick and made a smoked turkey cigar.
Availability: Supermarkets

* Turkey
Tom-Toms Turkey Snacks Stick Original
Wellshire Farms
877-467-2331 www.wellshirefarms.com
Bottom Line: 50 calories per serving (1 stick)
Details: One Yummy Hunter says she goes out Friday nights for happy hour with the gang and brings these tasty snacks so she won't be tempted to hit on the bar snacks. The only downside is that now she's feeding everyone at the bar. *Helen:* Delicious turkey taste! *Eric:* I'm trying to figure out how to make a sandwich out of these things.
Availability: Online

* Turkey Bologna
Applegate Farms, Turkey Bologna
Applegate Farms
866-587-5858 www.applegatefarms.com
Bottom Line: 70 calories per serving (2 oz)
Details: Baloney-loving Yummy Hunters are thrilled to discover this is as good as the original. *Helen:* I've been hooked on this since our Yummy Hunters wrote in about it. *Eric:* No baloney. You gotta try it.
Availability: Health food stores; store locations and ordering online

* Veggie Pizza Pepperoni
Yves, Veggie Cuisine, Veggie Pizza Pepperoni
Hain Celestial Group, Inc.
800-667-9837 www.yvesveggie.com
Bottom Line: 70 calories per serving (16 slices)
Details: Yummy Hunters take a pita bread, spread tomato sauce, light mozzarella and Veggie Pizza Pepperoni on top, and they have a delicious homemade pizza. *Helen & Eric:* We can vouch for the Yummy Hunters' recipe—it was delish.
Availability: Health food stores and ordering online at www.thegoodlunch.com

We're the country that has more food to eat than any other country in the world . . . . and more diets to keep us from eating it.

MEALS
Lunch & Dinner

As DIETERS, we dream of the perfect meal. More often than not, those dreams go unfulfilled and we chase after food for the rest of the day. Thanks to our Yummy Hunters' selections, our dreams will now come true.

---

* Asian Noodles
Amy's, Asian Noodles, Stir-Fry
Amy's Kitchen, Inc.
707-578-7188 www.amyskitchen.com
Bottom Line: 240 calories per serving (10 oz)
Details: Yummy Hunters tell us it tastes like lo mein, which is taboo on any diet. *Helen & Eric:* We're lo mein lovers, too. The noodles have a great Asian flavor, and the veggies are fresh and delicious.
Availability: Health food stores, many supermarkets, some club stores; store locations online and ordering at www.nomeat.com

Beef with Raisins and Olives
Ethnic Gourmet, Picadillo, Beef with Raisins and Olives
Hains Celestial Group, Inc.
800-434-4246 www.ethnicgourmet.com
Bottom Line: 340 calories per serving (10 oz)
Details: Yummy Hunters tell us how much they enjoy the exotic spices. Others who don't allow themselves to eat beef because of the high calories say this is worth the splurge. *Eric:* The sweet raisins combine with the hot spices to create an intriguing blend of flavors.
Availability: Supermarkets and heath foods stores

Broccoli and Cheddar Baked Potato
Weight Watchers, Smart Ones, Broccoli and Cheddar Baked Potato
Heinz Frozen Food Company
800-762-0228 www.weightwatchers.com
Bottom Line: 260 calories per serving (10 oz)
Details: Yummy Hunters rave this is one special potato and say this cheesy duo really hits the spot at lunch. *Helen:* Delicious broccoli and cheddar combo. The potato was cooked to perfection. *Eric:* This spud's for us!
Availability: Supermarkets

Broccoli and Cheese
Barber Foods, Light, Stuffed Chicken Breasts, Broccoli and Cheese, Chicken
Barber Foods
800-577-2595 www.barberfoods.com
Bottom Line: 220 calories per serving (1 piece)
Details: *Eric:* This is another of Helen's fabulous finds. She discovered it in her local supermarket, served it to her kids with a side of brown rice and it was a huge success. *Helen:* My daughter has lost 30 pounds, and this chicken dish is one of the reasons her diet has been so successful.
Availability: Supermarkets, some health food stores and Wal-Mart

Brown Rice & Vegetables
Amy's, Brown Rice & Vegetables Bowl
Amy's Kitchen, Inc.
707-578-7188 www.amyskitchen.com
Bottom Line: 250 calories per serving (10 oz)
Details: Vegetarian Yummy Hunters who have problems with their weight say this great-tasting low-calorie food fills them up and is a fabulous find. One enjoys the fact this frozen meal uses brown instead of white rice. *Helen & Eric:* Tasty blend of veggies, tofu and brown rice make this one enjoyable bowl.
Availability: Health food stores, many supermarkets, some club stores; store locations online and ordering at www.nomeat.com

Caesar, Grilled Chicken Wraps
Kraft, South Beach Diet, Grilled Chicken Caesar Wraps
Kraft Foods, Inc.
800-932-7800 www.krafthealthyliving.com
Bottom Line: 230 calories per serving (1 pckg)
Details: Yummy Hunters just found this in their local supermarkets and are loving the convenience as well as the taste. *Helen:* Great take-along lunch. Everything is wrapped separately and all you have to do is make it and eat it! *Eric:* How cool is this!
Availability: Supermarkets

Cheese
Amy's Cheese Lasagna
Amy's Kitchen, Inc.
707-578-7188 www.amyskitchen.com
Bottom Line: 380 calories per serving (10.3 oz)
Details: Yummy Hunters confess most low-cal lasagnas are watery; however, this is really perfect. The cheese isn't rubbery and the sauce is delicious. *Helen & Eric:* We think it's the big cheese, too.
Availability: Health food stores, many supermarkets, some club stores; store locations online and ordering at www.nomeat.com

Cheese Pizza
Amy's, Cheese Pizza in a Pocket Sandwich
Amy's Kitchen, Inc.
707-578-7188 www.amyskitchen.com
Bottom Line: 300 calories per serving (4½ oz)
Details: Yummy Hunters just have to recommend this tasty and convenient product. One raves her 12-year-old daughter, who continually watches her weight, adores these pocket sandwiches and when she eats them doesn't feel like she's on a diet. *Helen:* We just popped it in the micro and it was done. *Eric:* Looks like a calzone, but when we bit into it, it was pizza through and through.
Availability: Health food stores, many supermarkets and some club stores; store locations online and ordering at www.nomeat.com

Cheese Shells
Healthy Choice, Stuffed Pasta Shells
ConAgra Foods, Inc.
800-457-6649 www.healthychoice.com
Bottom Line: 290 calories per serving (11.15 oz)
Details: Yummy Hunters give this an A+ for flavor.
Another adds these shells have an authentic
Italian restaurant taste. *Helen:* Oh, my God!
Cheesy goodness stuffed into a perfect pasta
shell. *Eric:* Helen just reminded me that just
because they're called stuffed pasta shells doesn't
mean that I have to stuff them in my mouth.
Helen: You needed me to tell you this?!
Availability: Supermarkets

✳ Chicken And Noodles
Shelton's, Chicken And Noodles
Shelton's Poultry, Inc.
800-541-1833 www.sheltons.com
Bottom Line: 170 calories per serving (1 cup)
Details: Yummy Hunters say it's a creamy comfort
on cold winter days. Another adds it's a perfect
kid dish. *Helen:* Tender noodles and chicken
swimming in a delicious, full-bodied sauce. *Eric:*
Wow, great sauce! I yammed it up in record time.
Availability: Health food stores and online

✳ Chicken & Vegetables
Weight Watchers, Smart Ones, Fire-Grilled Chicken & Vegetables
H.J. Heinz Company
800-762-0228 www.weightwatchers.com
Bottom Line: 280 calories per serving (283 g)
Details: Yummy Hunters say this is a favorite and
one they can splurge on. Another says when
cooking something high in calories for her family,
which she won't eat, she microwaves this
delicious dish for herself and doesn't feel
deprived. *Helen:* A really nice change from the
boring chicken dieters constantly complain about.
Eric: Chicken and veggies are done to perfection.
Availability: Supermarkets

✳ A Low-Fat Product

∗ Chicken Chow Mein
La Choy, Chicken Chow Mein
ConAgra Foods, Inc.
800-338-8831 www.lachoy.com
Bottom Line: 110 calories per serving (1 cup)
Details: *Helen:* This is Eric's find. He's always enjoyed it; he just never knew it was low-cal. He tells me it reminds him of the Chinese food he ate as a kid. *Eric:* Even if you're sharing, this is a humongous amount of great-tasting food. Now, don't get me wrong, I'm not saying you have to share.
Availability: Supermarkets

Chicken Massaman
Ethnic Gourmet, Chicken Massaman
Hains Celestial Group, Inc.
800-434-4246 www.ethnicgourmet.com
Bottom Line: 330 calories per serving (12 oz)
Details: Yummy Hunters love this dish because it enables them to have exotic Thai food in a portion-controlled meal. *Helen*: Set your taste buds afire with this delicious Thai favorite. *Eric:* Massaman, that must mean SPICYMAN! So spicy I had to call a bomb disposal unit.
Availability: Supermarkets and health food stores

∗ Chicken Mediterranean
Stouffer's, Lean Cuisine, Café Classics, Chicken Mediterranean
Nestlé USA, Inc.
800-993-8625 www.leancuisine.com
Bottom Line: 240 calories per serving (10½ oz)
Details: Yummy Hunters who diet and live alone say it's easy for them to take this portion-controlled meal and pop it into the microwave. They're surprised and delighted this meal tastes so good. *Helen:* Tender chicken, tasty veggies and perfect pasta all in a delicately seasoned sauce. *Eric:* Gourmet-tasting meal that gave me another reason to enjoy chicken.
Availability: Supermarkets; store locations online

Chicken Parmigiana
Healthy Choice, Chicken Parmigiana
ConAgra Foods, Inc.
800-457-6649 www.healthychoice.com
Bottom Line: 320 calories per serving (11 oz)
Details: *Helen:* I was in line at my local grocery store and noticed a lady buying six of these dinners. I asked if they were on sale. She laughed and said, "Honey, I eat these every night and I've lost 15 pounds." They're the most authentic-tasting chicken parms I've ever had. *Eric:* We needed to experience this Italian delight for ourselves and were every bit as thrilled. So, break out the checkered tablecloths.
Availability: Supermarkets

Chicken Tandoori with Spinach
Ethnic Gourmet, Chicken Tandoori with Spinach
Hains Celestial Group, Inc.
800-434-4246 www.ethnicgourmet.com
Bottom Line: 330 calories per serving (11 oz)
Details: Yummy Hunters rave this dish is exotically delicious. *Helen:* We mixed the rice in with the chicken and, together with the spinach and blend of spices, it made for a delicious meal. *Eric:* The real deal. The kick will send you all the way to New Delhi.
Availability: Supermarkets and health food stores

* Chicken with Almonds
Stouffer's, Lean Cuisine, Café Classics, Chicken with Almonds
Nestlé USA, Inc.
800-993-8625 www.leancuisine.com
Bottom Line: 260 calories per serving (8½ oz)
Details: Yummy Hunters who eat chicken when dieting rave this dish is the best. They chirp about its true Asian punch. *Helen:* Tender chicken with an oriental flair. We love those almonds! *Eric:* I really did enjoy the sauce and I'm always conflicted as to whether I should pick the almonds out and eat them separately or eat them together with the chicken. So delicious, this bird flew off the plate.
Availability: Supermarkets; store locations online

Chili, Cornbread
Amy's, Chili and Cornbread Whole Meal
Amy's Kitchen, Inc.
707-578-7188 www.amyskitchen.com
Bottom Line: 340 calories per serving (1 meal)
Details: Yummy Hunters say it has just the right amount of spice and rave the corn bread is fluffy and tasty. *Helen:* Hard to believe this deliciously filling meal can be on anyone's diet! *Eric:* This delightful duo creates a satisfying and tasty Mexican meal.
Availability: Health food stores, supermarkets and some club stores; store locations online and ordering at www.nomeat.com

Eggplant, Three Bean
Celentano, Eggplant Wraps with Three Bean Filling
Celentano Food Products, Inc.
888-767-4621 www.rosina.com
Bottom Line: 220 calories per serving (10 oz)
Details: Yummy Hunters tell us that the most frustrating thing when they're dieting is to finish a meal and still be hungry. They say the beans in this tasty meal fill them up. *Helen:* I hear you. When I'm full after a meal, I'm less likely to eat something I'm not supposed to. *Eric:* The eggplant was tender and the bean filling flavorful. Out of this world! Bean me up, Scotty!
Availability: Supermarkets and health food stores

* Enchilada with Black Beans and Vegetables
Amy's, Black Bean Vegetable Enchilada
Amy's Kitchen, Inc.
707-578-7188 www.amyskitchen.com
Bottom Line: 170 calories per serving (1 enchilada)
Details: Yummy Hunters love the blend of veggies and black beans. One who has lost 20 pounds says she's happy that she's never had to give up on her beloved enchiladas. *Helen:* I recommend one for lunch and two for dinner. *Eric:* I have no self-control, so it's dos, amigos.
Availability: Supermarkets and health food stores

Enchilada with Cheese
Amy's, Cheese Enchilada
Amy's Kitchen, Inc.
707-578-7188 www.amyskitchen.com
Bottom Line: 220 calories per serving (4.75 oz)
Details: Yummy Hunters say it tastes like it comes from a Mexican restaurant. They have to be careful and eat only one for lunch or else they're fasting the rest of the day! *Helen:* Thank God Eric shared this with me; otherwise, I would have gobbled both up and sent my calorie count into the stratosphere. *Eric:* Anything I can do to help . . .
Availability: Supermarkets, health food stores and some club stores; store locations online

* Glazed Turkey Tenderloins
Stouffer's, Lean Cuisine, Café Classics, Glazed Turkey Tenderloins
Nestlé USA, Inc.
800-993-8625 www.leancuisine.com
Bottom Line: 260 calories per serving (9 oz)
Details: Yummy Hunters say the turkey is tender and extremely tasty and makes them yearn for Thanksgiving. *Helen:* The turkey was phenomenal, but the potatoes weren't especially tasty. *Eric:* So we made a big mush and it was delicious.
Availability: Supermarkets; store locations online

Indian Nattar Paneer
Amy's, Indian Nattar Paneer
Amy's Kitchen, Inc.
707-578-7188 www.amyskitchen.com
Bottom Line: 320 calories per serving (10 oz)
Details: Yummy Hunters declare they often need something different at mealtime and this fun and filling Indian dish fits their diet plan. *Helen:* We agree, variety is the spice of dieting and this mouth-watering dish has that and more. *Eric:* Kudos to Amy's Kitchen for bringing a taste of India to my kitchen.
Availability: Health food stores, supermarkets and some club stores; store locations online and ordering at www.nomeat.com

* A Low-Fat Product

Macaroni & Cheese
Seeds of Change, Macaroni & Cheese
Master Foods USA™
888-762-4240 www.seedsofchange.com
Bottom Line: 420 calories per serving (11 oz)
Details: Yummy Hunters say it delivers that great mac and cheese taste they've grown up loving.
Helen: Creamy, tasty and delightful! *Eric:* Reminds me of the wonderful mac and cheese I got as a kid from Horn & Hardart here in New York. For those who don't know, this was a self-service automat and a place that still wells deeply in my heart.
Availability: Health food stores; store locations online and ordering at www.netgrocer.com

Macaroni and Cheese
Stouffers, Lean Cuisine, Everyday Favorites, Macaroni and Cheese
Nestlé USA, Inc.
800-993-8625 www.leancuisine.com
Bottom Line: 300 calories per serving (10 oz)
Details: Yummy Hunters say when they plan their meals in advance they have more dieting success. They add this is one of their top cheesy choices.
Helen: This mac 'n cheese is a low-calorie choice. The sauce may be lighter, but the flavor is still big. We had it one night for dinner and found we were still a little hungry. So, we make it one of our lunchtime favorites. *Eric:* On the other hand, you can have three for dinner. *Helen:* Aren't you on a diet? *Eric:* How about two?
Availability: Supermarkets; store locations online

* Mexican Tamale Pie
Amy's, Mexican Tamale Pie
Amy's Kitchen, Inc.
707-578-7188 www.amyskitchen.com
Bottom Line: 150 calories per serving (8 oz)
Details: Yummy Hunters say if they're going to have a big dinner, this is a great lunch choice.
Helen: Eric's been known to eat two at one sitting. *Eric:* I confess—send me south of the border!
Availability: Supermarkets and health food stores

Mushroom
Thai Kitchen, Rice Noodle Bowl, Mushroom
Epicurean International, Inc.
800-967-8424 www.thaikitchen.com
Bottom Line: 120 calories per serving (1 cup prepared)
Details: Yummy Hunters say it has a nice harmony of Asian flavors and is very satisfying and delicious. *Helen & Eric:* We break out the chopsticks for this conveniently delicious, take-along meal.
Availability: Supermarkets, health food stores and online

Palak Paneer
Amy's, Palak Paneer
Amy's Kitchen, Inc.
707-578-7188 www.amyskitchen.com
Bottom Line: 240 calories per serving (142 g)
Details: Yummy Hunters say now they have another way to enjoy the taste of India. *Helen:* Indian food at its very best. *Eric.* Full of exotic flavor, very filling and saved me a trip to the Indian restaurant where I would have overeaten.
Availability: Health food stores, supermarkets and some club stores; store locations online

Penne Pollo
Weight Watchers, Smart Ones, Bistro Selections, Penne Pollo
Heinz Frozen Food Company
800-762-0228 www.eatyourbest.com
Bottom Line: 290 calories per serving (10 oz)
Details: Yummy Hunters enjoy the creamy mixture of flavors. *Helen:* This delicious sauce transforms an ordinary pasta meal into an extraordinary dining experience. *Eric:* Very tender and well-seasoned chicken on top of a delicious-tasting and perfectly cooked pasta. This was a real treat because frozen pasta can come out mushy. I ate this faster than you can say "me amore."
Availability: Supermarkets

Penne with Roasted Vegetables
Celentano, Penne with Roasted Vegetables
Celentano Food Products, Inc.
888-767-4621 www.rosina.com
Bottom Line: 230 calories per serving (10 oz)
Details: Yummy Hunters who've tried to cut down on their meat are happy to find delicious alternatives, and this is one of their favorites. *Helen:* Italian vegetables roasted to perfection in a delicious-tasting tomato sauce. Another outstanding pasta meal and, oh, how filling. *Eric:* This penne is penne perfect.
Availability: Supermarkets and health food stores

* Ravioli, Cheese
Annie's Cheesy Ravioli
Annie's Homegrown
781-224-9639 www.annies.com
Bottom Line: 180 calories per serving (1 cup)
Details: Yummy Hunters love the convenience of this easy take-along can. One Yummy Hunter says she can eat it right out of the can without heating it, it's so good. *Helen:* I always thought ravioli was taboo for dieters, but this portion-controlled can has made a believer out of me. *Eric:* Cheesy ravioli in a rich, tasty and cheesy tomato sauce.
Availability: Supermarkets and health food stores; online and ordering at www.netgrocer.com

* Rice and Red Beans
Goya, Rice and Red Beans
Goya Foods, Inc.
201-348-4900 www.goya.com
Bottom Line: 160 calories per serving (¼ cup)
Details: Yummy Hunters say it's great to get away from meat and chicken, and this supplies variety to their dieting menu needs. *Helen & Eric:* We found we needed a triple serving to make it a satisfying meal. At a 160 calories, it makes for a great side dish. Add a little salsa for some extra fun.
Availability: Supermarkets and ordering online at www.netgrocer.com

Risotto with Eggplant, Tofu and Spinach
Celentano, Risotto with Eggplant, Tofu and Spinach
Celentano Food Products, Inc.
888-767-4621 www.rosina.com
Bottom Line: 340 calories per serving (10 oz)
Details: Yummy Hunters say they'll do anything to make dieting easier, and when something as convenient and delicious as this Celentano product comes along, they are delighted beyond words. *Helen:* The creamy tofu and spinach mix complements the firm mushrooms and makes this the perfect risotto. *Eric:* What a delicious and tasty combination. These people are artistes!
Availability: Supermarkets and health food stores

Roasted Garlic Chicken
Stouffer's, Lean Cuisine, Café Classics, Roasted Garlic Chicken
Nestlé USA, Inc.
800-993-8625 www.leancuisine.com
Bottom Line: 200 calories per serving (8⅞ oz)
Details: Yummy Hunters tell us the chicken portion is tasty and filling. One declares when she comes home from work, she puts it in her microwave and swears that the only time the dog begs at the table is when she smells that garlic aroma. *Helen & Eric:* The subtle but tasty garlic flavor complements the moist chicken.
Availability: Supermarkets; store locations online

Salisbury Steak
Stouffer's, Lean Cuisine, Dinnertime Selections, Salisbury Steak
Nestlé USA, Inc.
800-993-8625 www.leancuisine.com
Bottom Line: 320 calories per serving (15½ oz)
Details: Yummy Hunters on low-carb diets confess they make this instead of potatoes. *Eric:* The steak and gravy are terrific, but I needed to put gravy on the potatoes for taste. I overcooked the veggies so watch them carefully.
Availability: Supermarkets; store locations and ordering online

Salisbury Steak, Vegetarian
Amy's, Country Dinner, Vegetarian Salisbury Steak
Amy's Kitchen, Inc.
707-578-7188 www.amyskitchen.com
Bottom Line: 390 calories per serving (312 g)
Details: Yummy Hunters rave this is a nice, healthy meal — great if you don't have the time or you don't want to make a meal from scratch. *Helen:* I don't eat beef, so this is a delicious alternative for me. *Eric:* Tastes like steak to me.
Availability: Health food stores, supermarkets and some club stores; store locations online

* Salmon
Stouffer's, Lean Cuisine, Spa Cuisine Classics, Salmon with Basil
Nestlé USA, Inc.
800-225-1180 www.leancuisine.com
Bottom Line: 260 calories per serving (9 ⅝-oz)
Details: Salmon-loving Yummy Hunters are overjoyed to finally find a salmon meal that is easy to make and tastes great. *Helen:* This low-fat meal makes for five-star dining in your very own kitchen. *Eric:* Worth opening a bottle of good white wine for this one.
Availability: Supermarkets; store locations online

Samosa Wraps
Amy's, Organic, Indian Samosa Wraps
Amy's Kitchen, Inc.
707-578-7188 www.amyskitchen.com
Bottom Line: 240 calories per serving (142 g)
Details: Yummy Hunters who eat many prepared meals rave about its unique flavor and consider it one of their favorites. *Helen:* Dieters beware! This package contains two servings. One is OK for a light lunch or dinner. If you're hungry, don't be tempted to go for a second — have a side salad instead. *Eric:* Be careful not to overcook or it will be on the dry side. Nicely seasoned.
Availability: Health food stores, supermarkets and some club stores; store locations online

Santa Fe Style, Rice and Beans
Weight Watchers, Smart Ones, Santa Fe Style, Rice and Beans

Heinz Frozen Food Company
800-762-0228 www.weightwatchers.com
Bottom Line: 300 calories per serving (10 oz)
Details: One Yummy Hunter confesses she's never enjoyed diet foods, but a coworker told her how wonderful this meal was and she became addicted. *Helen:* Delightful sauce tops off this hearty dish. *Eric:* Viva la Mexican madness!
Availability: Supermarkets

* Shells & White Cheddar
Annie's, Organic, Macaroni & Cheese

Annie's Homegrown
781-224-9639 www.annies.com
Bottom Line: 370 calories per serving (1 cup prepared)
Details: *Eric:* This is one of my finds and it's unbelievable. The instructions say the best way to prepare it is to use butter and skim milk, but I used olive oil. The shells were tender; the cheddar cheese as fresh and tasty as if I had cut it from a deli chunk. *Helen:* I shared it with my son and daughter and we cleaned our plates.
Availability: Supermarkets and health food stores; online and ordering at www.netgrocer.com

* Shepherd's Pie
Amy's, Shepherd's Pie

Amy's Kitchen, Inc.
707-578-7188 www.amyskitchen.com
Bottom Line: 160 calories per serving (227 g)
Details: Yummy Hunters don't miss the meat in this hearty shepherd's pie. They especially like the potato crust and chunky vegetables. *Helen:* This low-fat vegetarian pie is a must for every dieter. One at lunch fills me up and warms my soul. *Eric:* Will someone direct me to Trafalgar Square.
Availability: Health food stores, supermarkets and some club stores; store locations online and ordering at www.nomeat.com

* Shrimp, Fried Rice
Gorton's, Shrimp Bowl, Fried Rice
Gorton's
800-222-6846 www.gortons.com
Bottom Line: 320 calories per serving (10½ oz)
Details: Yummy Hunters who love fried rice declare this is their favorite lunch. They add that the shrimp are big enough not to get lost in the rice. *Helen:* But wait, I'm eating fried rice! I'm never allowed to eat fried rice on my diet. An incredible find! It tastes like the fried rice I remember eating at my local Chinese restaurant as a kid. *Eric:* When you wish upon a rice bowl . . .
Availability: Supermarkets

* Shrimp, Stir-Fry
Contessa, Shrimp Stir-Fry
Contessa Food Products
888-832-8000 www.contessa.com
Bottom Line: 140 calories per serving (8 oz)
Details: Yummy Hunters say after a hard day at work, this meal is a blessing; it takes just 10 minutes from freezer to dinner table. The family has a delicious hot meal and Yummy Hunters stay on their diet. *Helen:* We ate the entire bag, which added up to 210 calories each. If you're really hungry, this is a great meal. *Eric:* Stir it up.
Availability: Supermarkets; store locations online

Shrimp & Angel Hair Pasta
Stouffer's, Cafe Classics, Shrimp & Angel Hair Pasta
Nestlé USA, Inc.
800-225-1180 www.leancuisine.com
Bottom Line: 240 calories per serving (283 g)
Details: Yummy Hunters say they are reeling with delight now they can have a rich-tasting shrimp and pasta dish without going off their diet plan. *Helen:* Delicate pasta topped with nice-sized and very tasty shrimp. *Eric:* Soft, tender and juicy shrimps in a tasty sauce. Worth a great bottle of white wine.
Availability: Supermarkets; store locations online

Southwestern Style Chicken Wraps
Kraft, South Beach Diet, Southwestern Style Chicken Wraps
Kraft Foods, Inc.
800-932-7800 www.krafthealthyliving.com
Bottom Line: 240 calories per serving (1 pckg)
Details: Yummy Hunters love the south-of-the-border flavor as much as the convenience. Another adds it's foods like this that make staying on a diet so easy. *Helen:* Just wrap it up. *Eric:* Wrap could have had a little more flavor, but the chicken was tasty and the salsa had a nice tangy kick.
Availability: Supermarkets

Spinach Feta
Amy's, Spinach Feta In A Pocket Sandwich
Amy's Kitchen, Inc.
707-578-7188 www.amyskitchen.com
Bottom Line: 250 calories per serving (128 g)
Details: Yummy Hunters find it convenient and very filling. They just mic it, and take it. *Helen:* Strong feta flavor, fresh-tasting spinach make this the perfect pocket sandwich. *Eric:* Perfect combo of cheese and spinach. Loved it.
Availability: Health food stores, supermarkets and some club stores; store locations online and ordering at www.nomeat.com

Sweet & Sour Chicken
Weight Watchers, Smart Ones, Sweet & Sour Chicken
H.J. Heinz Company
800-762-0228 www.weightwatchers.com
Bottom Line: 150 calories per serving (255 g)
Details: Yummy Hunters tell us how fresh tasting and delicious this dish is. Others say it enables them to have this restaurant favorite without any guilt. They also say the low calories leave room for them to have a little steamed rice with it. *Helen:* My restaurant favorite, guilt free! You can't beat that! *Eric:* Sauce makes it for me. Juicy chicken, not too sweet, just right.
Availability: Supermarkets

Thai, Stir-Fry
Amy's, Thai, Stir-Fry
Amy's Kitchen, Inc.
707-578-7188 www.amyskitchen.com
Bottom Line: 310 calories per serving (9½ oz)
Details: Yummy Hunters say it's exotically delicious.
Helen: Great balance of savory tastes and textures.
Eric: Not only does Amy capture the flavors of
faraway lands, she keeps the calorie count from
flying away. Amy, do you make house calls?
Availability: Health food stores, supermarkets and
some club stores; store locations online and
ordering at www.nomeat.com

Three Cheese Stuffed Rigatoni
**Stouffer's, Lean Cuisine, Café Classics Bowl, Three
Cheese Stuffed Rigatoni**
Nestlé USA, Inc.
800-993-8625 www.leancuisine.com
Bottom Line: 260 calories per serving (10 oz)
Details: Yummy Hunters rave how good this dish
is. *Helen:* Ingenious the way they stuff the little
rigatonis. You get a cheesy taste with every bite!
Eric: I'm an opera lover, so nothing goes better
with Rigoletto than these rigatonis. Boy, do I love
to hear those high cheeses!
Availability: Supermarkets; store locations and
ordering online

Tofu Scramble
Amy's, Tofu Scramble in a Pocket Sandwich
Amy's Kitchen, Inc.
707-578-7188 www.amyskitchen.com
Bottom Line: 180 calories per serving (4 oz)
Details: Yummy Hunters eat these Tofu Scrambles
in the car on the way to the gym and it gives them
all the breakfast they need. Others love 'em any
time of day. *Helen:* Tasty and moist egglike filling
surrounded by a crisp sandwich. *Eric:* So unique,
convenient and tasty you'll be scrambling to the
store for this one.
Availability: Supermarkets and health food stores

Turkey Breast, Roasted
Stouffer's, Lean Cuisine, Dinnertime Selections, Roasted Turkey Breast
Nestlé USA, Inc.
800-993-8625 www.leancuisine.com
Bottom Line: 340 calories per serving (396 g)
Details: Yummy Hunters love the Thanksgiving taste of this dinner any time of the year. *Helen:* Turkey was tender, veggies were great. *Eric:* Cornbread stuffing was terrific!
Availability: Supermarkets; store locations online

Vegetable Lasagna
Amy's, Vegetable Lasagna
Amy's Kitchen, Inc.
707-578-7188 www.amyskitchen.com
Bottom Line: 300 calories per serving (9½ oz)
Details: Yummy Hunters say they gobble it up at 5:30 PM and never have to nosh all evening. *Helen & Eric:* If we were stranded on a desert island, this would be one of our picks.
Availability: Health food stores, supermarkets and some club stores; store locations online and ordering at www.nomeat.com

Vegetable Loaf
Amy's, Veggie Loaf Whole Meal
Amy's Kitchen, Inc.
707-578-7188 www.amyskitchen.com
Bottom Line: 280 calories per serving (10 oz)
Details: Vegetarian Yummy Hunters jokingly declare this is a "meat and potatoes" kind of meal. *Helen:* Very filling, very satisfying. We especially liked the peas and corn. The mashed potatoes were like Momma used to make. *Eric:* Our kind of comfort food.
Availability: Health food stores, supermarkets and some club stores; store locations online and ordering at www.nomeat.com

Food for thought has no calories.

MUFFINS

MUFFINS are the highest point on which you can layer a glob of strawberry jam. So, there!

✳ Blueberry
Duncan Hines, Kellogg's All-Bran Muffins, Blueberry
Duncan Hines
800-362-9834 www.duncanhines.com
Bottom Line: 140 calories per serving prepared (¼ cup mix)
Details: Yummy Hunters say it's like having cake for breakfast, but without the guilt! Even if they double the recipe, it's still only 4 points on Weight Watchers. *Helen:* 280 calories per muffin and don't dream about getting more than six out of that box unless you like minis. *Eric:* Blueberries add a delicate sweetness to this delicious muffin.
Availability: Supermarkets

✳ Blueberry Corn
Nutritious Creations Fat Free, Blueberry Corn Muffin
Nutritious Creations, LTD
631-666-9815 www.bakedgoods.tv
Bottom Line: 120 calories per serving (2 oz)
Details: Yummy Hunters say they would never suspect it's a low-calorie, fat-free muffin, it's that good. They keep a bunch in the fridge and mic them on high for 30 seconds and they're in heaven. *Helen:* Great-tasting corn muffin with sweet blueberries throughout. *Eric:* Just eat and enjoy.
Availability: Some health food stores, delis and online

✱ Bran Muffin
Hodgson Mill, Bran Muffin Mix
Hodgson Mill, Inc.
800-525-0177 www.hodgsonmill.com
Bottom Line: 130 calories per serving prepared (¼ cup dry)
Details: Yummy Hunters love the taste of bran. They say you can make a batch and freeze what you don't eat because they're just as fresh out of the microwave later. *Helen:* When I baked these, I threw in a handful of raisins for a little extra spice. *Eric:* One was very filling, so we don't think you need to double up on the recipe.
Availability: Supermarkets and online

✱ Chocolate Chip
Soybran, Chocolate Chip Muffin Mix
Twins Food Industries, Inc.
800-895-9994 www.twinsfood.com
Bottom Line: 154 calories per serving (1 muffin)
Details: *Helen:* I discovered these at a fitness conference and the sweet taste of chocolate (you know I love chocolate) got my attention before my taste buds began to explore the hearty bran flavor. *Eric:* More kudos to Helen. We think you'll want what the manufacturer calls a Texas-sized muffin, which means doubling up the recipe.
Availability: Online

✱ Cinnamon Raisin
Health Valley, Fat Free, Cinnamon Raisin, Scones
Hain Celestial Group, Inc.
800-423-4846 www.hain-celestial.com
Bottom Line: 180 calories per serving (1 scone)
Details: Yummy Hunters say these scones remind them of their childhood and they remember how nice it is to diet with an old favorite. *Helen:* These scones make a quick and easy breakfast or a filling in-between snack. *Eric:* So good, these scones will gather no moss.
Availability: Supermarkets, health food stores and ordering online at www.leesmarket.com, www.naturemart.com and www.netgrocer.com

Corn
Chatila's, New Generation, Corn Muffins
Chatila's Bakery
877-619-5398 www.chatilasbakery.com
Bottom Line: 70 calories prepared (1 muffin)
Details: One Yummy Hunter says she will drive anywhere to get a good muffin. Lucky for her the bakery was only one state away. She rates this corn muffin with the best of any homemade ones she's every had. *Helen:* We toasted ours and put some Get Healthy America Raspberry preserve on it and it made for one sweet treat. *Eric:* One bite and you'll be singing Chatila to the tune of "Cecilia" by Simon and Garfunkel.
Availability: Online

* Corn
Hodgson Mill, Corn Bread and Muffin Mix
Hodgson Mill, Inc.
800-525-0177 www.hodgsonmill.com
Bottom Line: 130 calories prepared (¼ cup dry)
Details: Yummy Hunters rave how really good it is. Doesn't need butter, just a little jelly and they're good to go. *Helen:* There is nothing like a hot corn muffin to excite your palate and delight your taste buds. We practically inhaled them after they were baked. *Eric:* You mustn't think too badly of us. Sometimes we just get carried away.
Availability: Some supermarkets, by phone and online

* Corn
Muffin Delite, Gourmet Diet Corn Toppers
Muffin Delite
800-604-8800
Bottom Line: 100 calories per serving (1 top)
Details: One Yummy Hunter insists the top of the muffin is the best part, and this one is tops. *Helen:* This is an ingenious product. First-class corn muffin taste. They made the best part of the muffin even better. *Eric:* Hats off to the bakers at Muffin Delite!
Availability: Supermarkets

* Deep Chocolate
Vita Muffin, Deep Chocolate, VitaTops
Vitalicious, Inc.
212-233-6030 www.vitalicious.com
Bottom Line: 100 calories per serving (1 muffin)
Details: Yummy Hunters say these muffins are great for eating breakfast on the go. They pop one in the toaster, add a little jam and they're out the door. *Helen:* Let's talk chocolate. This rich, chocolatey flavor will not disappoint even the hardest hard-core chocaholics. *Eric:* Enough talking, let the eating begin.
Availability: Supermarkets, health food stores, online and at www.gethealthyamerica.com

Double Chocolate Chip
Muffins n More, Double Chocolate Chip
Honig Food Corp.
718-302-5955
Bottom Line: 80 calories per serving (1 muffin)
Details: Chocaholic Yummy Hunters came up for air long enough to drop us a line about these Yummy muffins. *Helen:* Sweet and decadent, everything a chocaholic fiend like me feeds on. *Eric:* I microwaved it and topped it off with some low-fat frozen yogurt and had a delicious muffin sundae.
Availability: Online at www.gethealthyamerica.com

* Multi Bran
Vita Muffin, Fat Free, Multi Bran
Vitalicious, Inc.
212-233-6030 www.vitalicious.com
Bottom Line: 100 calories per serving (½ muffin)
Details: Yummy Hunters say it gives them some real get-up-and-go. Dieters' choice when they don't want anything overly sweet for breakfast, and it makes them feel like they've had a good start to the day. *Helen:* We microwaved it for 30 seconds and it came out oven-fresh and delicious. *Eric:* You know how hard it is to wait 30 seconds when you are overwhelmed by the aroma of these delicious muffins? Do you?
Availability: Online at www.gethealthyamerica.com

Oat Bran
Chatila's, New Generation, Oat Bran Muffins
Chatila's Bakery
877-619-5398 www.chatilasbakery.com
Bottom Line: 60 calories prepared (1 muffin)
Details: Our "drive-anywhere" Yummy Hunter says this muffin is low-carb, has no fat, is high in fiber and loaded with taste, making it the very best muffin she's ever had. *Helen:* I had to look twice at the label because this is one delicious muffin. *Eric:* I'm still singing Chatila!
Availability: Online

* Oatbran
Muffins n More, Gourmet Diet Muffins, Oat Bran
Honig Food Corp.
718-302-5955
Bottom Line: 80 calories per serving (2¼ oz)
Details: Yummy Hunters say so, so easy. They just pop them into the microwave and out come delicious, homemade—like, oat bran-flavored muffins. *Helen:* Light and not too sweet make these muffins irresistible. *Eric:* I knew there was a reason I scarfed them down in record time. Just be careful you don't burn your tongue!
Availability: Online at www.gethealthyamerica.com

* Spice
Soybran, Spice Muffin Mix
Twins Food Industries, Inc.
800-895-9994 www.twinsfood.com
Bottom Line: 121 calories prepared (1 muffin)
Details: *Helen:* Another flavor by the same company that I discovered at a fitness conference. The indescribably wonderful taste brings something new and different to breakfast. *Eric:* Spice is nice, so we think you'll want to double the size.
Availability: Online

Before you eat it, Scotch tape it to your thighs and see how it looks.

NUTS

Our Yummy Hunters have come up with a variety of nuts that would drive any squirrel crazy. However, we are not squirrels, we are dieters, so watch those portion sizes and don't go nuts over nuts.

BBQ, Soybeans
Chambers Farms, Tosteds, Big Barn BBQ
Chambers Farms
888-527-9296 www.tosted.com
Bottom Line: 138 calories per serving (⅓ cup)
Details: Yummy Hunters love the BBQ flavor. This product satisfies their cravings for nuts while enabling them to eat many more nuts for the calories. *Helen:* Goodbye peanuts, hello soy nuts. *Eric:* Big BBQ taste makes me nuts for these nuts.
Availability: Online

* Mesquite Barbeque
Amaizing Corn, Mesquite Barbeque Nuts
Dakota Gourmet
800-727-6663 www.dakotagourmet.com
Bottom Line: 100 calories per serving (1-oz bag)
Details: Yummy Hunters who watch their calories watch their intake of nuts, but they make room for these special treats. *Helen & Eric:* Real gourmet flavor, which lends itself to slowly savoring each nut.
Availability: Health food stores, some vending machines, by phone and online

Slightly Spicy
Grandpa Po's, Nutra Nuts, Slightly Spicy
Nutra Nuts, Inc.
323-260-7457 www.nutranuts.com
Bottom Line: 160 calories per serving (⅓ cup)
Details: These unique popcorn-based products
that crunch like a nut fascinate Yummy Hunters.
They say when watching their weight, these are
nice alternative to nuts. One Yummy Hunter
measures out her third of a cup and it takes a while
to eat. *Helen & Eric:* We were completely blown
away by this new and exciting snack. With three
great flavors, there's something for everyone.
Availability: Some health food stores; store
locations and ordering online

Sun Flower Seeds
Frito Lay, Sun Flower Seeds, Seed Only
Frito-Lay, Inc.
800-352-4477 www.fritolay.com
Bottom Line: 180 calories per serving (3 tbsp)
Details: Yummy Hunters say they need to keep
themselves busy when dieting and nothing works
better than eating sunflower seeds, one by one
and savoring each bite. *Helen & Eric:* Who eats one
at a time! Let's face it, if God wanted us to eat one
at a time, he wouldn't have given us the ability to
scoop up a handful and shove it into our mouths.
Availability: Supermarkets

✳ Sweet & Sour Green Soybeans
Eat Your Heart Out, Sweet & Sour Green Soybeans
Eat Your Heart Out
201-333-3077 www.eatyourheartoutsnacks.com
Bottom Line: 90 calories per serving (.74-oz bag)
Details: *Helen:* I first tasted the dried peaches at a
spa and enjoyed them so much I contacted the
manufacturer to get its other products. These
soybeans are a totally unique and delicious
product. *Eric:* Another reason everyone should go
to a health spa. Also available in Indian Spice.
Availability: Online

Unsalted, Soybeans
Chambers Farms, Tosteds, Unsalted
Chambers Farms
888-526-9296 www.tosted.com
Bottom Line: 140 calories per serving (⅓ cup)
Details: Yummy Hunters like to measure out their portions, take them to work and then munch on them throughout the day. *Helen:* Lovely soy flavor makes these beans irresistible. *Eric:* Subtle, but addictive taste.
Availability: Online

Those who indulge, bulge.

PANCAKES & WAFFLES

YOU MIGHT THINK there is no sweeter or more treacherous start to the dieter's day than sitting down before a plate of pancakes or waffles. Wrong! Our Yummy Hunters have discovered the most delicious low-calorie pancakes and waffles that will satisfy even the nondieter's palate. How sweet it is!

---

* Blueberry
Kashi's, Go Lean, Blueberry Frozen Waffles
Kashi Company
858-274-8870 www.kashi.com
Bottom Line: 170 calories per serving (2 waffles)
Details: Yummy Hunters say these waffles are satisfying and quick to make. An easy hot breakfast and not their ordinary ho-hum meal. *Helen & Eric:* We couldn't agree more. We think these waffles will be popping up all over!
Availability: Supermarkets and health food stores

* Buckwheat
Up Country, Organics, Buckwheat Pancake & Waffle Mix
B & G Foods, Inc.
800-525-2540 www.upcountryorganics.com
Bottom Line: 80 calories per serving (⅓ cup dry)
Details: When our Yummy Hunters discovered this product, they went pancake happy. They tell everyone how they eat pancakes everyday and still stay on their diet. *Helen & Eric:* Not as fluffy as ordinary pancakes, but they have a wonderfully sweet taste.
Availability: Supermarkets, health food stores and online at www.mybrandsinc.com

* Cinnamon Apple
Vermont Gold, Cinnamon Apple, Pancake Mix
Vermont Gold
888-556-2753 www.vermontgoldusa.com
Bottom Line: 80 calories per serving (⅓ cup prepared)
Details: Yummy Hunters embrace this product because it puts the pancake back into their breakfast. They add it reminds them of the apple pancakes their dad used to make before Sunday church services. *Helen:* The sweetness of apple bread. We were floored! *Eric:* I can't get over how something this good could be in anybody's diet.
Availability: Online and at www.leesmarket.com

* Multigrain
Up Country, Organics, Buckwheat Pancake & Waffle Mix
B & G Foods, Inc.
800-525-2540 www.upcountryorganics.com
Bottom Line: 80 calories per serving (⅓ cup dry)
Details: Yummy Hunters joyously say that thanks to this product they can now enjoy a once forbidden breakfast meal that they loved as children. *Helen & Eric:* A must for anyone who loves pancakes.
Availability: Supermarkets, health food stores and online at www.mybrandsinc.com

* Original
Up Country, Organics, Buckwheat Pancake & Waffle Mix
B & G Foods, Inc.
800-525-2540 www.upcountryorganics.com
Bottom Line: 40 calories per serving (⅓ cup dry)
Details: Yummy Hunters love the basic pancake taste and never feel guilty eating it for breakfast or with a little ice cream on top for a deliciously satisfying snack. *Helen:* Classic pancake taste. Makes up fluffy and delicious. Everything a pancake should be. *Eric:* Calling all dieters—time to put pancakes back on the menu.
Availability: Supermarkets, health food stores and ordering online at www.mybrandsinc.com

* A Low-Fat Product

✳ Plain
Aunt Jemima, Low Fat, Frozen Pancakes
The Quaker Oats Co.
800-417-2247 www.auntjemima.com
Bottom Line: 190 calories per serving (3 pancakes)
Details: Yummy Hunters rave about the convenience of these traditional pancakes. It makes a dieter's breakfast fun, and now Yummy Hunters scream for joy. *Helen:* We stuffed them with jelly and made jellyrolls. *Eric:* We made sure the windows were closed before we screamed for joy.
Availability: Supermarkets and online

✳ Plain
Eggo Frozen Waffles
Kellogg Co.
877-993-4467 www.kellogg.com
Bottom Line: 140 calories per serving (2 waffles)
Details: Yummy Hunters like these basic waffles with syrup. One says she's lost 47 pounds, but she "never had to let go of her Eggos." *Helen & Eric:* Kudos to our Yummy Hunter for her inspiring weight loss! These waffles will fit as nicely into your diet plan as they will into the toaster.
Availability: Supermarkets

✳ Whole Wheat, Buttermilk
Hodgson Mill, Whole Wheat, Buttermilk, Pancake Mix
Hodgson Mill, Inc.
800-525-0177 www.hodgsonmill.com
Bottom Line: 120 calories per serving (⅓ cup dry)
Details: Our Yummy Hunters like the whole wheat flavor and rave about how easy this mix is to make. Others served them as a dessert with fresh fruit and a little Cool Whip. *Helen & Eric:* We sliced bananas in ours; nothing beats the warmth of fresh pancakes.
Availability: Supermarkets, health food stores, by phone and online

It takes a minute to eat and months to take off.

PIZZA

LET'S TALK PIZZA. Dieters used to have only two choices. Get rid of the cheese by burying it in the bottom of a garbage pail so it couldn't be reattached; or get rid of the bread, which you could bury in the same way. Now, thanks to our Yummy Hunters, picks, you can keep your pizza in one piece.

Cheese Pizza
Amy's, Cheese Pizza in a Pocket Sandwich
Amy's Kitchen, Inc.
707-578-7188 www.amyskitchen.com
Bottom Line: 300 calories per serving (4½ oz)
Details: Yummy Hunters just have to recommend this tasty and convenient product. One raves her 12-year-old daughter, who continually watches her weight, adores these pocket sandwiches and when she eats them doesn't feel like she's on a diet.
Helen: We just popped it in the micro and it was done. *Eric:* Looks like a calzone, but when we bit into it, it was pizza through and through.
Availability: Health food stores, supermarkets and some club stores; store locations online and ordering at www.nomeat.com

5-Cheese
Red Barron Stuffed Pizza Slices
Red Barron
800-769-7980 www.redbarron.com
Bottom Line: 310 calories per serving (1 piece)
Details: Pizza-crazy Yummy Hunters say this baby is just stuffed with flavor. *Helen:* Use caution— you could easily eat two slices without taking a breath. *Eric:* Now you tell me!
Availability: Supermarkets

Mexican
Health Is Wealth, Mexican Pizza
Val Vasilef, Health Is Wealth Products, Inc.
856-728-1998 www.healthiswealthfoods.com
Bottom Line: 330 calories per serving (1 piece)
Details: Yummy Hunters say this Mexican-inspired pizza is a welcome change from a traditional pizza. *Helen:* Dieters can rejoice. There are now so many delicious low-calorie choices that will fit easily into any diet plan. *Eric:* Break out the sombrero for this true-to-life Mexican Quesadilla pizza à la Health Is Wealth.
Availability: Supermarkets and health food stores

Mushroom & Spinach
Linda McCartney, Mushroom & Spinach Pizza
H.J. Heinz Company
888-474-3175 www.linda-mccartney.com
Bottom Line: 320 calories per serving (½ pizza)
Details: Yummy Hunters who are fans of Linda are excited to find this delicious product. Others comment how tasty it is and like the fact the company donates all proceeds to the Make A Wish Foundation. *Helen:* Fresh-tasting mushrooms and spinach layered on a crispy crust. *Eric:* We also tried spicy Thai, and it was wickedly good.
Availability: Supermarkets and health food stores

* Pizza
Campbell's, Soup at Hand, Pizza
Campbell Soup Company
800-257-8443 www.campbellsoup.com
Bottom Line: 140 calories per serving (1 container)
Details: Yummy Hunters say it's pizza on the go and wonder what they will think of next. One adds that getting full for 130 calories is a real treat. *Helen:* Rich-flavored soup for a cold winter's day. Although it didn't taste like pizza to us, it had a very appealing smoky flavor. *Eric:* No, we didn't overcook it!
Availability: Supermarkets and ordering online at www.netgrocer.com

Roasted Vegetable
Amy's, Roasted Vegetable Pizza
Amy's Kitchen, Inc.
707-578-7188 www.amyskitchen.com
Bottom Line: 270 calories per serving (⅓ pie)
Details: Yummy Hunters tell us their college-aged kids love the fact there's no fattening cheese and they think the glazed onions are out of sight. Yummy Hunter parents stock up and send their kids care packages. *Helen:* Great combination of veggies on top of a delicious crust. *Eric:* Our eyes are glazed over from these sweet, glazed onions.
Availability: Supermarkets and health food stores

Roasted Vegetable Pizza
Stouffer's, Cafe Classics, Roasted Vegetable Pizza
Nestlé USA, Inc.
800-225-1180 www.leancuisine.com
Bottom Line: 330 calories per serving (170 g)
Details: One Yummy Hunter says her kids give her high-fives for serving them. Others love the convenience of just popping them in the micro and having themselves a tasty and filling meal. *Helen:* Crispy crust with fresh-tasting vegetables on top. So exciting to see another delicious-tasting, low-cal pizza on the market. *Eric:* I gave myself a high-five after eating this winner.
Availability: Supermarkets; store locations online

Spinach
Amy's, Spinach Pizza
Amy's Kitchen, Inc.
707-578-7188 www.amyskitchen.com
Bottom Line: 310 calories per serving (⅓ pie)
Details: Yummy Hunters tell us they don't like pizza that's heavy on the sauce, so this is just right for them. They say one-third of this cheesy, spinachy gem satisfies their appetites and dieting desires. *Helen & Eric:* Rich, cheesy flavor with tasty spinach, a hint of tomatoes and a crunchy whole wheat crust. What else could you ask for?
Availability: Supermarkets and health food stores

Spinach & Mushroom Pizza
Stouffer's, Cafe Classics, Spinach & Mushroom Pizza
Nestlé USA, Inc.
800-225-1180 www.leancuisine.com
Bottom Line: 310 calories per serving (173 g)
Details: Yummy Hunters love this Weight Watchers
6-point, deep-dish delight. *Helen & Eric:* Alfredo
sauce topping with fresh-tasting spinach and
mushrooms make this a must.
Availability: Supermarkets; store locations online

Tomato & Basil
Morningstar Farms, Veggie, Pizza Burgers, Tomato & Basil
Kellogg Co.
800-557-6525 www.morningstarfarms.com
Bottom Line: 130 calories per serving (1 burger)
Details: Yummy Hunters say this is another food to
help them stay on their diets. They add it has a
superb pizza taste and it's the perfect choice when
they want something quick and easy. *Helen & Eric:*
We gobbled them up like kids, washing them down
with a nice tall glass of Mistic Wild Cherry.
Availability: Supermarkets

✱ Veggie Pizza
Dr. Praeger's, Veggie Pizza Burgers
Ungar's Food Products
201-703-1300 www.drpraegers.com
Bottom Line: 120 calories per serving (1 burger)
Details: Yummy Hunters say this is the ultimate
pizza burger. *Helen:* This is what you get when you
cross the perfect veggie burger with the ultimate
pizza seasoning. *Eric:* This is one doctor that knows
how to doctor-up a great veggie burger.
Availability: Some supermarkets and store
locations online

*Too many people confine their exercise to
jumping to conclusions, running up bills,
stretching the truth, bending over backward,
lying down on the job, sidestepping responsibility
and pushing their luck.*

POPCORN

Wɪᴛʜ ғᴏᴏᴅ, ᴛʜᴇʀᴇ ɪs ɴᴏ ɢʀᴇᴀᴛᴇʀ emotional connection than popcorn to movies. Plus, it's dark in the theater and no one can see how much you're shoveling in your mouth. So, if you love movies or just love eating in the dark, these selections will satisfy the urge for crunch. With all the new and exotic flavors, popcorn has become one of our favorite palate pleasers.

Butter Licious
Jolly Time Butter Licious Light
American Pop Corn Company
712-239-1232 www.jollytime.com
Bottom Line: 130 calories per serving (5 cups popped)
Details: Yummy Hunters say it's as good as movie house popcorn and can't believe this buttery delight is on their diet plans. *Helen:* I don't usually like to put butter on my popcorn. However, I liked this popcorn because I didn't find the butter to be overwhelming. *Eric:* I agree—just enough butter to give it a nice sweet flavor.
Availability: Online

✱ Caramel
Go Lightly, Sugar Free, Caramel Popcorn
Hillside Candy
800-524-1304 www.hillsidecandy.com
Bottom Line: 90 calories per serving (¾ cup)
Details: Yummy Hunters say every bit as good as Cracker Jacks. Satisfies their sweet tooth cravings more than regular popcorn. *Helen:* Crunchy popcorn with a sweet caramel coating that's just thick enough. *Eric:* The prize is in the taste.
Availability: Supermarkets, drug stores and ordering online at www.jambsupply.com

Chocolate Cashew Almond Popcorn
Harry and David, Sugar Free, Moose Munch
Harry and David
877-322-1200 www.harryanddavid.com
Bottom Line: 120 calories per serving (1 oz)
Details: Yummy Hunters rave about this popcorn and say it gives them so many different and delicious taste sensations. Another raves she can't believe this is on anyone's diet. *Helen:* Crunchy popcorn covered with rich chocolate, cashews and almonds makes this outstanding in every way. *Eric:* I would like to adopt Harry and David. Better still, I want them to adopt me so I can live with them in their factory.
Availability: Harry and David locations and online

* Kettle Korn
Orville Redenbacher's, Smart Pop, 94% Fat Free, Kettle Korn
ConAgra Foods, Inc.
800-457-6649 www.orville.com
Bottom Line: 140 calories per serving (7 cups popped)
Details: One Yummy Hunter told us she discovered Kettle Korn at a local street fair and it was love at first bite. *Helen:* Sweet, crunchy and utterly delicious. *Eric:* They've taken the smell of popcorn to an even sweeter level. Why didn't someone think of this product sooner? How sweet it is!
Availability: Supermarkets

* Kettle Korn
Pure Snax, Original Kettle Corn
Hain Celestial Group, Inc.
800-434-4246 www.hainspuresnax.com
Bottom Line: 120 calories per serving (1½ cups)
Details: Yummy Hunters say this delicious popcorn offers them salt, sweetness and crunchiness all rolled into one. *Helen:* I measured out a cup and a half and had me a lot of sweet crunch. Amen! *Eric:* I love when Helen gets religion. But I'd love it more if she shared more of the popcorn with me.
Availability: Supermarkets and health food stores

✱ Light
Herr's, Light Popcorn
Herr Foods, Inc.
610-932-9330 www.herrs.com
Bottom Line: 120 calories per serving (3 cups)
Details: Yummy Hunters say that when dieting, they need to feel they can eat something in large amounts. They measure their three cups, sometimes even six, and are thrilled to have enough to munch on for hours. *Helen:* Light and crunchy with just the right amount of salt. *Eric:* Crunch, crunch, crunch!
Availability: Supermarkets in the Northeast and online

Nut and Honey
LesserEvil, Bee Nutty!, Nut and Honey
Lesserevil, Inc.
914-779-3000 www.lesserevil.com
Bottom Line: 120 calories per serving (1¼ cups)
Details: Yummy Hunters like to buy the 2.5-ounce bag and take it with them to the office. One bag keeps them snacking all afternoon. *Helen:* The sweetness of honey turns this popcorn into an extraordinary treat. *Eric:* Don't forget the nuts!
Availability: Supermarkets, health food stores and online

✱ Olive Oil
Good Health, Half Naked Pop Corn With A Hint Of Olive Oil
Good Health Natural Foods, Inc.
631-261-5608 www.e-goodhealth.com
Bottom Line: 120 calories per serving (4 cups)
Details: Yummy Hunters tell us when they're dieing they measure four cups out and they can crunch all afternoon without going back into the kitchen. One adds she sneaks a bag into the movies and enjoys the treat without guilt. *Helen:* The hint of olive oil gives this popcorn a unique gourmet taste. *Eric:* The naked truth is that half naked is delish!
Availability: Supermarkets, health food stores and online

White Cheddar
Smart Food, White Cheddar Reduced Fat Popcorn
Frito-Lay
800-352-4477 www.fritolay.com
Bottom Line: 140 calories per serving (3 cups)
Details: Yummy Hunters praise the super cheddar taste and buy the large bag for parties and the individuals for themselves. *Helen & Eric:* Warning: We opened the large bag and ate the whole thing.
Availability: Supermarkets, drugstores and health food stores

Each day I try to enjoy something from each of the four food groups: the bonbon group, the salty snack group, the caffeine group and the whatever-the-thing-in-the-tinfoil-in-the-back-of-the-fridge-is group.

✽ A Low-Fat Product

POULTRY

Rᴏᴀsᴛ ɪᴛ, sᴛᴜғғ ɪᴛ, ɢʀɪɴᴅ ɪᴛ, dice it, barbeque it or marinate it; poultry done right is always tender and delicious. It better be, because no matter how you slice it, unless you're a vegetarian, you're going to be eating chicken or turkey four or five times a week.

Artichoke & Garlic Smoked Turkey and Chicken
Aidells, Artichoke & Garlic Sausage, Smoked Turkey and Chicken
Aidells Sausage Co.
877-243-3557 www.aidells.com
Bottom Line: 160 calories per serving (1 link)
Details: Yummy Hunters love the original and tasty combination of ingredients. They add they love it with pasta or on steamed spinach when they're watching their carbs. *Helen & Eric:* We sliced it and put it on Baker Honey Whole Wheat sandwich buns, with a little Grey Poupon and some romaine—yum!
Availability: Upscale grocery stores; store locations and ordering online

Broccoli and Cheese
Barber Foods, Light, Stuffed Chicken Breasts, Broccoli and Cheese, Chicken
Barber Foods
800-577-2595 www.barberfoods.com
Bottom Line: 220 calories per serving (1 piece)
Details: *Eric:* This is another of Helen's fabulous finds. She discovered it in her local supermarket, served it to her kids with a side of brown rice and it was a huge success. *Helen:* My daughter has lost 30 pounds, and this chicken dish is one of the reasons her diet has been so successful.
Availability: Supermarkets, some health food stores and Wal-Mart

Caesar, Grilled Chicken Wraps
Kraft, South Beach Diet, Grilled Chicken Caesar Wraps
Kraft Foods, Inc.
800-932-7800 www.krafthealthyliving.com
Bottom Line: 230 calories per serving (1 pckg)
Details: Yummy Hunters just found this in their local supermarkets and are loving the convenience as well as the taste. *Helen:* Great take-along lunch. Everything is wrapped separately and all you have to do is make it and eat it! *Eric:* Cool!
Availability: Supermarkets

Chicken
Casual Gourmet, Smoked Apple, Chicken Sausage
Casual Gourmet Foods, Inc.
727-298-8307 www.cgfoods.com
Bottom Line: 110 calories per serving (3 oz)
Details: Yummy Hunters tell us this delicious-tasting sausage has become a family favorite. They add smell is so important when preparing their food and the sweet aroma of this smoked apple sausage is just not to be believed. *Helen:* The standard by which all sausages should be judged. *Eric:* Also available in Mild Italian, Sweet Red Pepper and Basil and from last year's *Yummy Hunter's Guide*: Sun Dried Tomato and Herbs. What are you waiting for, run to the supermarket!
Availability: Supermarkets

* Chicken, Black Beans
Shelton's, Free Range, Mild, Chicken Chili with Black Beans
Shelton's Poultry, Inc.
800-541-1833 www.sheltons.com
Bottom Line: 210 calories per serving (1 cup)
Details: Yummy Hunters like this hearty, tasty dish and recommend adding low-fat sour cream for a bit of Mexican flair. *Helen:* Because I don't eat meat, this is a very tasty alternative when I'm in the mood for chili. *Eric:* We like the convenience of the can, the chili's robust flavor and the delicious chili— black bean combo.

Availability: Health food stores and online

* Chicken And Noodles
Shelton's, Chicken And Noodles
Shelton's Poultry, Inc.
800-541-1833 www.sheltons.com
Bottom Line: 170 calories per serving (1 cup)
Details: Yummy Hunters say it's a creamy comfort on cold winter days. Another adds it's a perfect kid dish. *Helen:* Tender noodles and chicken swimming in a delicious, full-bodied sauce. *Eric:* Wow, great sauce! I yammed it up in record time.
Availability: Health food stores and online

* Chicken & Vegetables
Weight Watchers, Smart Ones, Fire-Grilled Chicken & Vegetables
H.J. Heinz Company
800-762-0228 www.weightwatchers.com
Bottom Line: 280 calories per serving (283 g)
Details: Yummy Hunters say this is a favorite and one they can splurge on. Another says when cooking something high in calories for her family, which she won't eat, she microwaves this delicious dish for herself and doesn't feel deprived. *Helen:* A really nice change from the boring chicken dieters constantly complain about. *Eric:* Chicken and veggies were done to perfection.
Availability: Supermarkets

* Chicken Chow Mein
La Choy, Chicken Chow Mein
ConAgra Foods, Inc.
800-338-8831 www.lachoy.com
Bottom Line: 110 calories per serving (1 cup)
Details: *Helen:* This is Eric's find. He's always enjoyed it; he just never knew it was low-cal. He tells me it reminds him of the Chinese food he ate as a kid. *Eric:* Even if you're sharing, this is a humongous amount of great-tasting food. Now, don't get me wrong, I'm not saying you have to share.
Availability: Supermarkets

Chicken Massaman
Ethnic Gourmet, Chicken Massaman
Hains Celestial Group, Inc.
800-434-4246 www.ethnicgourmet.com
Bottom Line: 330 calories per serving (12 oz)
Details: Yummy Hunters love this dish because it enables them to have exotic Thai food in a portion-controlled meal. *Helen:* Set your taste buds afire with this delicious Thai favorite. *Eric:* Massaman, that must mean SPICYMAN! So spicy I had to call a bomb disposal unit.
Availability: Supermarkets and health food stores

✱ Chicken Mediterranean
Stouffer's, Lean Cuisine, Café Classics, Chicken Mediterranean
Nestlé USA, Inc.
800-993-8625 www.leancuisine.com
Bottom Line: 240 calories per serving (10½ oz)
Details: Yummy Hunters who diet and live alone say it's easy for them to take this portion-controlled meal and pop it into the microwave. They're surprised and delighted this meal tastes so good. *Helen:* Tender chicken, tasty veggies and perfect pasta all in a delicately seasoned sauce. *Eric:* Gourmet-tasting meal that gave me another reason to enjoy chicken.
Availability: Supermarkets; store locations online

Chicken Parmigiana
Healthy Choice, Chicken Parmigiana
ConAgra Foods, Inc.
800-457-6649 www.healthychoice.com
Bottom Line: 320 calories per serving (11 oz)
Details: *Helen:* I was in line at my local grocery store and noticed a lady buying six of these dinners. I asked if they were on sale. She laughed and said, "Honey, I eat these every night and I've lost 15 pounds." They're the most authentic-tasting chicken parms I've ever had. *Eric:* We needed to experience this Italian delight for ourselves and were every bit as thrilled. So, break out the checkered tablecloths.

Availability: Supermarkets

Chicken Tandoori with Spinach
Ethnic Gourmet, Chicken Tandoori with Spinach
Hains Celestial Group, Inc.
800-434-4246   www.ethnicgourmet.com
Bottom Line: 330 calories per serving (11 oz)
Details: Yummy Hunters rave this dish is exotically delicious. *Helen:* We mixed the rice in with the chicken and, together with the spinach and blend of spices, it made for a delicious meal. *Eric:* The real deal. The kick will send you all the way to New Delhi.
Availability: Supermarkets and health food stores

✳ Chicken with Almonds
Stouffer's, Lean Cuisine, Café Classics, Chicken with Almonds
Nestlé USA, Inc.
800-993-8625   www.leancuisine.com
Bottom Line: 260 calories per serving (8½ oz)
Details: Yummy Hunters who eat chicken when dieting rave this dish is the best. They chirp about its true Asian punch. *Helen:* Tender chicken with an oriental flair. We love those almonds! *Eric:* I really did enjoy the sauce and I'm always conflicted as to whether I should pick the almonds out and eat them separately or eat them together with the chicken. So delicious, this bird flew off the plate.
Availability: Supermarkets; store locations online

✳ Glazed Turkey Tenderloins
Stouffer's, Lean Cuisine, Café Classics, Glazed Turkey Tenderloins
Nestlé USA, Inc.
800-993-8625   www.leancuisine.com
Bottom Line: 260 calories per serving (9 oz)
Details: Yummy Hunters say the turkey is tender and extremely tasty and makes them yearn for Thanksgiving. *Helen:* The turkey was phenomenal, but the potatoes weren't especially tasty. *Eric:* So we made a big mush and it was delicious.
Availability: Supermarkets; store locations online

✳ Honey Roasted & Smoked Turkey
Tyson, Self-Serve Deli Meats, Honey Roasted & Smoked Turkey Breast
ConAgra Foods, Inc.
800-457-6649 www.healthychoice.com
Bottom Line: 60 calories per serving (4 slices)
Details: Yummy Hunters tell us that the smoked flavor really packs a punch! One adds it to a chopped salad with her own low-fat honey mustard dressing and says it's sensational. *Helen:* Turkey with a sweet, smoky flavor. We tried it on pita bread with a few pickles. It made a smoky, pickle-packin' sandwich. *Eric:* Try to say that 10 times fast.
Availability: Supermarkets

✳ Mesquite Turkey
Healthy Choice, Mesquite Turkey Breast
ConAgra Foods, Inc.
800-457-6649 www.healthychoice.com
Bottom Line: 60 calories per serving (4 slices)
Details: Yummy Hunters say this is a new and exciting way to eat turkey. One puts four slices on a slice of whole wheat bread and melts a piece of low-fat American cheese on top. *Helen:* Mild flavor with a subtle mesquite taste makes for a gourmet lunch meat. *Eric:* Give your lunch a kick with this Wild West sensation.
Availability: Supermarkets

Penne Pollo
Weight Watchers, Smart Ones, Bistro Selections, Penne Pollo
Heinz Frozen Food Company
800-762-0228 www.eatyourbest.com
Bottom Line: 290 calories per serving (10 oz)
Details: Yummy Hunters enjoy the creamy mixture of flavors. *Helen:* This delicious sauce transforms an ordinary pasta meal into an extraordinary dining experience. *Eric:* Very tender and well-seasoned chicken on top of a delicious-tasting and perfectly cooked pasta. This was a real treat because frozen pasta can come out mushy. I ate this faster than you can say "me amore."

Availability: Supermarkets

* Pesto Chicken
Casual Gourmet, Pesto, Chicken Sausages
Casual Gourmet Foods, Inc.
727-298-8307 www.cgfoods.com
Bottom Line: 120 calories per serving (3 oz)
Details: Yummy Hunters declare this has great sausage taste with less fat. They add it is a wonderful complement to spaghetti. *Helen:* We put it on a light bun with sautéed onions and a little mustard and it was delicious. *Eric:* Pesto adds a gourmet flavor without overwhelming the chicken. So, what came first, the chicken or the sausage?
Availability: Supermarkets

Roasted Chicken
Tyson, Roasted Chicken, Thighs
Tyson Foods, Inc.
800-233-6332 www.tyson.com
Bottom Line: 150 calories per serving (1 piece without skin)
Details: Yummy Hunters who love dark meat rave about this product. *Helen:* Even without the skin, the flavor comes through. This is so convenient we may never cook a chicken again. *Eric:* For someone who doesn't cook, this is heaven-sent.
Availability: Supermarkets

Roasted Garlic Chicken
Stouffer's, Lean Cuisine, Café Classics, Roasted Garlic Chicken
Nestlé USA, Inc.
800-993-8625 www.leancuisine.com
Bottom Line: 200 calories per serving (8⅞ oz)
Details: Yummy Hunters tell us the chicken portion is tasty and filling. One declares when she comes home from work, she puts it in her microwave and swears that the only time the dog begs at the table is when she smells that garlic aroma. *Helen & Eric:* The subtle but tasty garlic flavor complements the moist chicken.
Availability: Supermarkets; store locations online

✻ Roasted Turkey
Applegate, Roasted Turkey Breast
Applegate Farms
866-587-5858 www.applegatefarms.com
Bottom Line: 50 calories per serving (2 oz)
Details: Yummy Hunters say they eat a lot of salads when they're dieting, and these tasty turkey breasts really complement their greens. *Helen:* Fresh turkey that tastes like it was just sliced off the bone. This is a wonderful addition to sandwiches and salads. *Eric:* I rolled a slice and spread some light mayo on.
Availability: Health food stores; store locations and ordering online

✻ Shredded Chicken with Taco Sauce
Old El Paso, Shredded Chicken with Taco Sauce
General Mills, Inc.
800-999-7427 www.oldelpaso.com
Bottom Line: 60 calories per serving (¼ cup)
Details: Yummy Hunters say this makes their dieting so easy. One loves Mexican food but doesn't eat it out because she's not sure what's in it, so this is her salvation. *Helen:* The quarter cup didn't sound filling to me. However, when I spread it on a taco shell with lettuce, it became a satisfying meal. *Eric:* I suffer from Mexican madness—I needed two tacos.
Availability: Supermarkets

✻ Smoked Turkey
Hillshire Farm, Deli Select, Thin Sliced, Smoked Turkey Breast
Sara Lee
800-328-2426 www.hillshirefarm.com
Bottom Line: 50 calories per serving (6 slices)
Details: Yummy Hunters who grew up eating cold cuts need their slice meats when dieting, and this smoked turkey breast is a great alternative. *Helen:* It has a lighter smoky taste than some of the others we've tried, but it could be because the slices were very thin. Nevertheless, still very tasty. *Eric:* Thin is good. I wrapped it around a carrot stick and made a smoked turkey cigar.

Availability: Supermarkets

✳ Smoked White Turkey
Ball Park, Fat Free, Smoked White Turkey Franks
Ballpark Brands
888-317-5867 www.ballparkfranks.com
Bottom Line: 45 calories per serving (1 frank)
Details: Yummy Hunters love the smoky, barbeque flavor. *Helen:* For 45 calories this is a really special find. We each had two franks with Boar's Head mustard and some Sabrett onions on top. It was amazingly filling and oh-so-tasty! *Eric:* Smokin' good!
Availability: Supermarkets

Southwestern Style Chicken Wraps
Kraft, South Beach Diet, Southwestern Style Chicken Wraps
Kraft Foods, Inc.
800-932-7800 www.krafthealthyliving.com
Bottom Line: 240 calories per serving (1 pckg)
Details: Yummy Hunters love the south-of-the-border flavor as much as the convenience. One adds it's foods like this that make staying on a diet so easy. *Helen:* Just wrap it up. *Eric:* Wrap could have had a little more flavor, but the chicken was tasty and the salsa had a nice tangy kick.
Availability: Supermarkets

✳ Sun Dried Tomato and Herb Chicken
Casual Gourmet, Sun Dried Tomato and Herb Chicken Sausage
Casual Gourmet Foods, Inc.
727-298-8307 www.cgfoods.com
Bottom Line: 110 calories per serving (3 oz)
Details: Yummy Hunters say they love sausages and this one has the right amount of seasoning. *Helen:* The sun-dried tomatoes add a zesty flavor to this gourmet sausage. One was extremely filling. *Eric:* There's nothing causal about how delicious this chicken sausage is.
Availability: Supermarkets

Sweet & Sour Chicken
Weight Watchers, Smart Ones, Sweet & Sour Chicken
H.J. Heinz Company
800-762-0228 www.weightwatchers.com
Bottom Line: 150 calories per serving (255 g)
Details: Yummy Hunters tell us how fresh tasting and delicious this dish is. Others say it enables them to have this restaurant favorite without any guilt. They also say the low calories leave room for them to have a little steamed rice with it. *Helen:* My restaurant favorite, guilt free! You can't beat that! *Eric:* Sauce makes it for me. Juicy chicken, not too sweet, just right.
Availability: Supermarkets

* Turkey
Applegate Farms, Natural, Uncured Turkey Hot Dogs
Applegate Farms
866-587-5858 www.applegatefarms.com
Bottom Line: 120 calories per serving (1 hot dog)
Details: For flavor and natural goodness, Yummy Hunters like these better than beef hot dogs. *Helen:* We split them down the middle and then melted fat-free cheese on top. *Eric:* They looked and smelled so good, we held off eating them for a good 10 seconds.
Availability: Health food stores; store locations and ordering online

Turkey
Perdue, Turkey Burgers
Perdue
800-473-7383 www.perdue.com
Bottom Line: 160 calories per serving cooked (1 burger)
Details: Yummy Hunters like the convenience. The premade patties go straight from freezer to grill and always taste great and make a meal the entire family enjoys. *Helen:* Nice to have a delicious, preseasoned, portion-controlled turkey burger. *Eric:* These Yummy burgers remove the guesswork at mealtime and make dieting easy.
Availability: Supermarkets

✳ Turkey

Tom-Toms Turkey Snacks, Stick Original

Wellshire Farms

877-467-2331 www.wellshirefarms.com

Bottom Line: 50 calories per serving (1 stick)

Details: One Yummy Hunter says she goes out Friday nights for happy hour with the gang and brings these tasty snacks along so she won't be tempted to hit on the bar snacks. The only downside is that now she's feeding all her friends at the bar. *Helen:* Delicious turkey taste! *Eric:* I'm trying to figure out how to make a sandwich out of these things.

Availability: Online

✳ Turkey Bacon

Applegate Farms, Uncured, Turkey Bacon

Applegate Farms

866-587-5858 www.applegatefarms.com

Bottom Line: 38 calories per serving (1 slice)

Details: Yummy Hunters swear it tastes better than bacon and comes without the guilt. *Helen:* Its wonderfully smoky aroma makes cooking it a joy. It's sure to enhance any meal. *Eric:* True smokehouse-turkey flavor that goes great with eggs or on a TBLT (Turkey, Bacon, Lettuce, & Tomato).

Availability: Health food stores; store locations and ordering online

✳ Turkey Bologna

Applegate Farms, Turkey Bologna

Applegate Farms

866-587-5858 www.applegatefarms.com

Bottom Line: 70 calories per serving (2 oz)

Details: Baloney-loving Yummy Hunters are thrilled to discover this is as good as the original. *Helen:* I've been hooked on this since our Yummy Hunters wrote in about it. *Eric:* No baloney. You gotta try this delicious turkey bologna.

Availability: Health food stores; store locations and ordering online

Turkey Breast, Roasted
Stouffer's, Lean Cuisine, Dinnertime Selections, Roasted Turkey Breast
Nestlé USA, Inc.
800-993-8625 www.leancuisine.com
Bottom Line: 340 calories per serving (396 g)
Details: Yummy Hunters love the Thanksgiving taste of this dinner any time of the year. *Helen:* Turkey was tender, veggies were great. *Eric:* Cornbread stuffing was terrific!
Availability: Supermarkets; store locations online

Dieting is a losing battle.

✱ A Low-Fat Product

PRETZELS

W<small>E CAN EITHER</small> let dieting woes twist us up like a pretzel, or we can eat a pretzel and twist away those pounds. So, grab one of our selections and give yourself a great carbo boost.

✱ Butter
Snyder's of Hanover, Butter Snaps
Distributed by Snyder's of Hanover, Inc.
800-233-7125 www.snydersofhanover.com
Bottom Line: 120 calories per serving (24 pretzels)
Details: Yummy Hunters tell us it's the buttery taste that really gives these pretzels a terrific flavor. *Helen & Eric:* Not sure we want to eat an entire serving, but we love the buttery taste so much; we did treat ourselves and had a few with coffee for breakfast.
Availability: Health food stores and some supermarkets; store locations and ordering online

✱ Cheddar
Frito Lay, Rold Gold, Cheddar Flavored Tiny Twists
Frito-Lay, Inc.
800-352-4477 www.fritolay.com
Bottom Line: 110 calories per serving (20 pretzels)
Details: One Yummy Hunter says whenever he needs a quick, low-fat snack he reaches for these. *Helen:* Cheddar flavor gives it a step up over ordinary pretzels. *Eric:* I can't stop eating them!
Availability: Supermarkets

Chocolate
Harry and David, Sugar Free Chocolate Pretzels
Harry and David
800-547-3033 www.harryanddavid.com
Bottom Line: 170 calories per serving (5 pretzels)
Details: Yummy Hunters say these are simply the most delicious chocolate pretzels they've ever had. *Helen:* Another great, gourmet product from Harry and David. A really special-tasting and crunchy pretzel covered in a rich chocolate outer layer. Delicious! *Eric:* Believe it or not, you won't miss the sugar. You'll be too busy licking the chocolate off your fingers.
Availability: Harry and David locations and online

* Chocolate
Herr's, Chocolate Flavored Pretzel Rod
Herr Foods, Inc.
800-523-5030 www.herrs.com
Bottom Line: 90 calories per serving (1 pretzel rod)
Details: Yummy Hunters tell us this chocolate-covered pretzel is the real deal and they cannot believe it's only 2 points on Weight Watchers. *Helen:* Rich chocolate. Crunchy pretzel. I can't believe it's only 2 points, either. *Eric:* So much chocolate you almost forget it's a pretzel.
Availability: Supermarkets in the Northeast, online and at www.gethealthyamerica.com

* Honey Wheat
Frito Lay, Rold Gold, Honey Wheat, Braided Pretzels
Frito-Lay, Inc.
800-352-4477 www.fritolay.com
Bottom Line: 110 calories per serving (8 pretzels)
Details: One Yummy Hunter e-mailed us from college to say her mom sends her these, and now her entire floor waits for more care packages to arrive. *Helen:* Our Yummy Hunter is right, one bite and you'll be hooked. *Eric:* Unfortunately, you can eat as many as you want, but you won't look college-age again.
Availability: Supermarkets

* Honey Wheat with Sesame Seeds
Harry's, Honey Wheat with Sesame Seeds
Hain Celestial Group, Inc.
800-434-4246 www.harryssnacks.com
Bottom Line: 100 calories per serving (1 pretzel)
Details: Yummy Hunters who prefer whole wheat products think this is one terrific-tasting pretzel. *Helen:* Crunchy and wheaty with a slight sweet taste. *Eric:* Try putting some spicy mustard on for a sweet-and-sour surprise.
Availability: Store locations and ordering online

* Pretzel
The Snack Factory, Pretzel Crisps
The Snack Factory
609-683-5400 www.pretzelcrisps.com
Bottom Line: 110 calories per serving (20 pretzels)
Details: One Yummy Hunter says the flat surface holds the perfect amount of any kind of spread. *Helen:* Nice texture and great taste. A uniquely creative product. *Eric:* Be the first on your block to make a triple-decker cracker/pretzel sandwich. I put Brummel & Brown Yogurt on the bottom and a piece of low-fat cheese on the top.
Availability: Supermarkets

* Pumpernickel and Onion
Snyder's of Hanover, Organic, Pumpernickel and Onion
Distributed by Snyder's of Hanover, Inc.
800-233-7125 www.snydersofhanover.com
Bottom Line: 120 calories per serving (14 pretzels)
Details: Yummy Hunters rave they love the taste so much, they can eat them plain or dip them in cheese sauce. *Helen:* This is one of Eric's favorite foods, and after managing to grab the bag from him, I can see why. If you love the taste of pumpernickel, try these onion-flavored wonders. *Eric:* I know this is not an excuse, but I can't help myself.
Availability: Health food stores and some supermarkets; store locations and ordering online

Sesame
Ener-G, Pretzel Rings, Sesame
Ener-G Foods, Inc.
800-331-5222 www.ener-g.com
Bottom Line: 140 calories per serving (20 pretzels)
Details: Yummy Hunters rave this is one fabulous-tasting pretzel. The sesame seeds add an entirely new taste dimension. *Helen:* Taste that is out of this world. *Eric:* Takes you where no pretzel has ever gone before.
Availability: Some health food stores and by phone; store locations and ordering online and at www.leesmarket.com

* Unsalted
Newman's Own, Unsalted Rounds
Newman's Own Organics by the Second Generation
www.newmansownorganics.com
Bottom Line: 110 calories per serving (8 pretzels)
Details: Yummy Hunters love the fact these don't have any salt, which means no water retention. *Helen & Eric:* Crunchy, flavorful and we don't miss the salt one bit!
Availability: Supermarkets, health food stores; store locations and ordering online and at www.leesmarket.com

Diet is die with a t.

SALAD DRESSINGS

OUR YUMMY HUNTERS give new meaning to the phrase *dressing for success*. They have culled the huge selection of low-cal dressings and managed to find those precious few that taste great. More great news: Many have revealed some very imaginative recipes. How can you top that?

Blue Cheese
Marie's, Lite, Chunky, Blue Cheese
Dean Foods
800-441-3321 www.maries.com
Bottom Line: 80 calories per serving (2 tbsp)
Details: Yummy Hunters who love blue cheese choose this for salads and baked potatoes and say it doesn't taste low-cal at all. *Helen:* Dip, dip, dip — on anything and everything. *Eric:* Just remember to wipe your mouth after dipping.
Availability: Supermarkets

∗ Caesar
Cardini's, Fat Free, Caesar Dressing
T. Marzetti Company
614-846-2232 www.marzetti.com
Bottom Line: 40 calories per serving (2 tbsp)
Details: Yummy Hunters rave about this product's taste. One tells us how she is known for her low-cal Caesar salads. She takes romaine, sprinkles on veggie Parmesan, measures out the Cardini's, tosses and serves with a few walnuts on top. Her friends ask for the recipe, but she won't tell. *Helen & Eric:* We followed our Yummy Hunter's recipe, and what a salad! No wonder her friends keep coming back for more.
Availability: Supermarkets and online

Caesar
Kraft, Light Done Right!, Golden Caesar
Kraft Foods, Inc.
800-847-1997 www.kraftfoods.com
Bottom Line: 70 calories per serving (2 tbsp)
Details: Yummy Hunters say this is truly "classic" in every way. One adds she loves to make a chicken Caesar salad using this dressing, a piece of grilled chicken breast and some low-fat croutons. *Helen:* I added some roasted red peppers and I loved it. *Eric:* At least Helen invited me over for lunch. Hail Caesar! And hail Helen!
Availability: Supermarkets

* Catalina
Kraft, Free, Catalina, Fat Free Dressing
Kraft Foods, Inc.
800-847-1997 www.kraftfoods.com
Bottom Line: 50 calories per serving (2 tbsp)
Details: Yummy Hunters tell us when making tuna, instead of mayo they use Catalina and it's a delicious alternative. One says she's on Weight Watchers Core Program and in the afternoon she snacks on half an avocado with Catalina dressing and this not only fills her, but she feels like she's eating a big no-no. *Helen:* Kraft has created a unique flavor unlike any other salad dressing. *Eric:* Had me California dreamin'.
Availability: Supermarkets

* Country Italian
Wish-Bone, Just 2 Good, Country Italian
Unilever
800-697-7887 www.wish-bone.com
Bottom Line: 30 calories per serving (2 tbsp)
Details: Yummy Hunters say it adds the perfect flavors to salads without adding a greasy taste. *Helen:* Just like the label says, it's Just 2 Good! We used it on salads, and it's also an amazing marinade for chicken. *Eric:* To paraphrase the song . . . just too good to be true . . . can't stop from pouring you . . .
Availability: Supermarkets

* Creamy Bacon
Walden Farms, Calorie Free, Creamy Bacon
Walden Farms, Inc.
800-229-1706 www.waldenfarms.com
Bottom Line: 0 calories per serving (2 tbsp)
Details: Yummy Hunters buy this because it has no carbs and no calories and they are delighted to find it has plenty—and they mean plenty—of taste. *Helen:* We loved the unique, smoky flavor, and you don't have to like bacon to enjoy it. We tried it on sliced tomatoes and onion. Yummy! *Eric:* It's too delicious not to have calories. I'm calling in the Calorie Police to investigate.
Availability: Supermarkets, health food stores and online

* Ginger
Jo's All Natural, Japanese, Ginger Dressing
The Magic Bean Company
718-384-7989 www.magicbean.com
Bottom Line: 60 calories per serving (2 tbsp)
Details: Yummy Hunters tasted this dressing and told us they felt like they were in a Japanese restaurant. *Helen:* Authentic Japanese taste. If you love ginger, and we do, you're going to love this dressing *Eric:* You know, I'm crazy for ginger. Smells great! Tastes even better. You can put it on anything. I do.
Availability: Health food stores and online

* Gingerly Vinaigrette
Annie's Naturals, Low Fat, Gingerly Vinaigrette
Annie's Naturals
800-434-1234 www.anniesnaturals.com
Bottom Line: 40 calories per serving (2 tbsp)
Details: Yummy Hunters who love ginger love this Gingerly Vinaigrette and use it on salads and as a marinade for fish. *Helen:* Another super salad dressing from Annie's. We think it adds a unique and delicious Oriental flair to any salad. *Eric:* Hooray! More delicious ginger!
Availability: Health food stores and ordering online at www.leesmarket.com

Honey Mustard
Maple Grove Farms of Vermont, Lite, Honey Mustard Dressing
B & G Foods, Inc.
800-525-2540 www.maplegrove.com
Bottom Line: 80 calories per serving (2 tbsp)
Details: Yummy Hunters declare it's not only delicious as a salad dressing, but it has a certain richness that makes it a terrific sauce over cooked salmon. *Helen:* We poured it over a salad made with grilled chicken, lettuce, tomato and onions. *Eric:* More honey mustard, please.
Availability: Supermarkets, online and ordering at www.leesmarket.com

* Italian
Wish-Bone, Fat Free, Italian
Unilever
800-697-7887 www.wish-bone.com
Bottom Line: 20 calories per serving (2 tbsp)
Details: Yummy Hunters share their recipe for a quick and low-cal side dish. They chop some sweet onions, add chickpeas and pour on the Wish-Bone. *Helen:* Great recipe! It also makes a great marinade for chicken. *Eric:* Be careful what you wish for. This delicious dressing makes wishes come true. *Helen:* I rubbed the bottle three times and I still don't see a Mercedes in my driveway.
Availability: Supermarkets

* Late Harvest Riesling Vinegar
Cuisine Perel, Late Harvest, Riesling Vinegar
Cuisine Perel
510-232-0343 www.cuisineperel.com
Bottom Line: 5 calories per serving (1 tbsp)
Details: Yummy Hunters love the sweet and captivating taste. They now enjoy more salads at mealtime and declare this has helped them to eat less. *Helen:* It has a savory and delicious taste that makes it stand out on its own. *Eric:* Imagine pouring a fine Riesling over your salad and you'll get an idea of how wonderful this vinegar is.
Availability: Online at www.gourmetcountry.com

✳ Oriental
Walden Farms, Calorie Free, Oriental
Walden Farms, Inc.
800-229-1706 www.waldenfarms.com
Bottom Line: 0 calories per serving (2 tbsp)
Details: One Yummy Hunter told us how a friend at the gym turned her on to this uniquely delicious dressing. Now she uses it to dress her salads and pastas and declares dieting is fun. *Helen & Eric:* Fun when dieting? What a great concept!
Availability: Supermarkets, health food stores and online

Peanut Salad
A Taste of Thai, Peanut Salad Dressing Mix
Andre Prost, Inc.
800-243-0897 www.atasteofthai.com
Bottom Line: 40 calories per serving (2 tbsp)
Details: Yummy Hunters who love Thai, and even those who don't, tell us this is a uniquely rich and flavorful dressing that doesn't overpower. *Helen:* We agree, terrific taste that only enhances but never overwhelms the taste buds. *Eric:* A taste of Thai to die for. Made an ordinary chopped salad really delicious. I just wish I had somebody to serve it to.
Availability: Supermarkets, health food stores; store locations and ordering online

✳ Raspberry Vinaigrette
Annie's Naturals, Low Fat, Raspberry Vinaigrette
Annie's Naturals
800-434-1234 www.anniesnaturals.com
Bottom Line: 35 calories per serving (2 tbsp)
Details: *Eric:* Helen discovered this delicious, light dressing and uses it to make her summer salads sweet. *Helen:* Don't limit yourself to summer. Raspberry Vinaigrette is delectable 12 months a year. *Eric:* She's absolutely right. This is one star that deserves a 12-month run.
Availability: Health food stores; store locations and ordering online and at www.leesmarket.com

Raspberry Walnut Vinaigrette
Ken's Steak House, Lite, Raspberry Walnut Vinaigrette
Ken's Foods, Inc.
800-645-5707 www.kensfoods.com
Bottom Line: 80 calories per serving (2 tbsp)
Details: One Yummy Hunter raves about the subtle combination of flavors. *Helen:* The flavor of walnuts adds a special taste to this wonderfully delicious dressing. *Eric:* They've taken oil and vinegar to new heights with this wonderful combo.
Availability: Supermarkets and online

* Sun Dried Apricot Vinegar
Cuisine Perel, Sun Dried, Apricot Vinaigrette
Cuisine Perel
510-232-0343 www.cuisineperel.com
Bottom Line: 14 calories per serving (1 tbsp)
Details: Yummy Hunters say they use it to give salads a fruity taste, and it's so full of flavor they never have to add oil. *Helen:* We poured it over some sliced cucumbers and had a delicious salad. *Eric:* Try this savory vinaigrette; you'll be writing in with your own delicious recipes.
Availability: Online at www.gourmetcountry.com

* Thousand Islands
Walden Farms, Calorie Free, Thousand Islands
Walden Farms, Inc.
800-229-1706 www.waldenfarms.com
Bottom Line: 0 calories per serving (2 tbsp)
Details: Yummy Hunters tell us they use this as a topping on their favorite sandwiches. Others add they make tomato and onion salads using this dressing and the results are wonderful. *Helen:* We really like the tomato and onion salad recipe. *Eric:* A thousand thanks for this Thousand Islands dressing!
Availability: Supermarkets, health food stores and online

I'm not fat, I'm just short for my weight.

SAUCES
GRAVY, SAUCES

Thank God for gravy and sauces; otherwise, we'd be choking on some flavorless foods. You'll notice many of the sauces have a tomato base; however, each is unique and has its own special quality. So get sauced!

GRAVY

✳ Roasted Turkey
Heinz, Fat Free, Roasted Turkey Gravy
H.J. Heinz Co.
888-472-8437 www.heinz.com
Bottom Line: 10 calories per serving (¼ cup)
Details: Yummy Hunters declare eating plain turkey without the skin is so bland and boring, but once they tried Heinz Roasted Turkey Gravy, their diet meals came alive. *Helen & Eric:* This gravy is terrific on turkey, vegetables and baked potatoes.
Availability: Supermarkets

SAUCES

✳ Caponata Eggplant
Victoria, Sicilian Caponata Eggplant Sauce
Victoria Packing Corp.
718-927-3000 www.victoriapacking.com
Bottom Line: 50 calories per serving (½ cup)
Details: Yummy Hunters say great taste and great caloric bargain. *Helen:* Full-bodied tomato sauce is sure to add life to your favorite pasta or to some steamed stringbeans. *Eric:* Great southern Italian taste experience.
Availability: Supermarkets and ordering online at www.newyorkflavors.com

✳ Curry
Chef Shaikh's, Mild, Curry Sauce
Palace Foods, Inc.
800-curry-4u www.palacefoods.com
Bottom Line: 45 calories per serving (¼ cup)
Details: One Yummy Hunter excitedly told us she
sautéed chicken breasts with this sauce and then
to top it off added fresh spinach. *Helen:* We tried
this recipe and it was delicious. A true Indian
experience. *Eric:* Hurry, get this delicious curry.
Availability: Supermarkets, health food stores and
online

✳ Garden Vegetable
Classico, Garden Vegetable Primavera
International Gourmet Specialties Companies
888-337-2420 www.classico.com
Bottom Line: 60 calories per serving (½ cup)
Details: Yummy Hunters tell us it's their secret
ingredient for pasta primavera. They heat the
sauce, add fresh peppers and zucchini and pour it
over pasta. They rave the aroma alone brings their
families running. *Helen:* We went veggie crazy and
added broccoli, celery and onions. *Eric:* Straight
from the jar, it was straight from heaven.
Availability: Supermarkets and ordering online at
www.netgrocer.com

✳ Mushroom & Ripe Olives
Classico, Mushroom & Ripe Olives
International Gourmet Specialties Companies
888-337-2420 www.classico.com
Bottom Line: 60 calories per serving (½ cup)
Details: One Yummy Hunter tells us a friend made
a dish with this sauce for dinner and assured her
she could eat a full portion size and it wouldn't
hurt her diet. She has been using it every since.
Helen: Chunks of fresh-tasting mushrooms and
olives make this a very tasty and unique sauce.
Eric: Olives give it a bite and make it delectably
delightful.
Availability: Supermarkets and ordering online at
www.netgrocer.com

✳ Nacho Cheese
Mrs. Renfro's, Nacho Cheese Sauce
Renfro's Foods, Inc.
800-332-2456 www.renfrofoods.com
Bottom Line: 30 calories per serving (2 tbsp)
Details: Yummy Hunters pour Mrs. Renfro's over whole wheat pasta and say it makes the most delicious mac and cheese. *Helen:* Just mic it and dip. We dipped chips, pretzels and veggies and had a blast. *Eric:* Nacho, nacho man. I want to be a nacho man!
Availability: Supermarkets, gourmet food shops and online

✳ Portabello Mushrooms
Delallo, Portabello Mushrooms With Sweet Peppers
George E. Delallo Co. Inc.
800-433-9100 www.delallo.com
Bottom Line: 35 calories per serving (¼ cup)
Details: Yummy Hunters say their families will accept no substitute. Another, of Italian descent, called it "Magnifico." *Helen:* Rich tomato flavor with chunky pieces of mushrooms and peppers. I'm not Italian, but I can say "Bona Mia!" *Eric:* Please, would somebody tell me how to say in Italian ,"So full of flavor, you can become catatonic with delight."
Availability: Online

✳ Puttanesca
Francis Coppola, Organic Puttanesca
Francis Coppola Brands
707-967-0442 www.mammarellafoods.com
Bottom Line: 50 calories per serving (½ cup)
Details: One Yummy Hunter says since going on her diet, the only thing that has saved her is this sauce. Another pours it over spaghetti squash instead of pasta. *Helen:* Fresh, rich ingredients that brighten up any pasta or chicken meal. *Eric:* Now I know what Paulie was serving to the Corleone soldiers when they "went to the mattresses."
Availability: Supermarkets, health food stores and online

✳ Red Clam
Progresso, Red Clam
General Mills, Inc.
800-200-9377 www.progressosoup.com
Bottom Line: 60 calories per serving (½ cup)
Details: Yummy Hunters love the flavor of Progresso Red Clam sauce, especially over spaghetti squash. *Helen:* The clams were plump and juicy. The tomato sauce was rich and flavorful. We poured it over whole wheat pasta. Terrific! *Eric:* I love a good linguini with clam sauce. I give this three clams up!
Availability: Supermarkets

✳ Spinach
Ethnic Gourmet, Punjab Saag Spinach Sauce
Hains Celestial Group, Inc.
800-434-4246   www.ethnicgourmet.com
Bottom Line: 50 calories per serving (4 oz)
Details: One Yummy Hunter tells us she followed the recipe on the label and had an incredibly delicious and filling low-cal meal. *Helen:* Ethnic taste at its best. I added extra spinach and it was fabulous. *Eric:* This is one saucy sauce.
Availability: Supermarkets and health food stores

✳ Tomato & Basil
Classico, Tomato & Basil
International Gourmet Specialties Companies
888-337-2420 www.classico.com
Bottom Line: 60 calories per serving (½ cup)
Details: One Yummy Hunter, whose husband had to go on a diet for medical reasons, declares this sauce helped him continue to enjoy his pasta. *Helen:* Rich tomato flavor and with just the right amount of basil. *Eric:* Bravissimo! Classico makes it terrifico!
Availability: Supermarkets and ordering online at www.netgrocer.com

The first thing you lose on a diet is your sense of humor.

SEASONINGS & SWEETENERS

FLAVORS, MARINADES, OILS, SEASONINGS,
SPICES, SWEETENERS

LET'S FACE IT, no matter how many delicious low-cal products our Yummy Hunters discover, there will always be a food product or recipe that needs a little sprucing up. So, all you readers, want to sweeten the pot, spice up the next book and generally butter us up? Send in your flavor favorites.

FLAVORS

* Butter
Butter Buds, Butter-Flavored Granules
Cumberland Packing Corp.
www.butterbuds.com
Bottom Line: 5 calories per serving (1 tbsp liquid)
Details: Yummy Hunters say they use this product as a melted butter substitute and can't tell the difference. *Helen:* Mixes easily with hot water and is great to pour over seafood or potatoes. I love to buy fresh lobsters and dunk 'em in Butter Buds. *Eric:* I can't wait for my invite.
Availability: Supermarkets and drugstores; store locations online and ordering at
 www.brooklynpremiumcorp.com

* Butter
I Can't Believe It's Not Butter, Spray
Unilever Best Foods
800-634-0302 www.tasteyoulove.com
Bottom Line: 0 calories per serving (5 sprays per topping)
Details: Yummy Hunters say they love it on baked potatoes and pasta and it tastes just like butter. *Helen & Eric:* We can't believe it's not butter, either.
Availability: Supermarkets

Get the latest info at **www.yummyhunters.com**   237

✳ Buttery
Smart Balance, Light, Buttery Spread
Heart Beat Foods
201-568-9300 www.smartbalance.com
Bottom Line: 45 calories per serving (1 tbsp)
Details: Yummy Hunters say besides loving the taste, this spread has no hydrogenated fat, so it makes their doctors very happy. *Helen:* We tried it on bread, crackers, even made eggs with it and it tastes and spreads like butter to us. *Eric:* Oh, the marvels of modern science!
Availability: Supermarkets

MARINADES

✳ Dijon and Honey
Lawry's, 30 Minute Marinade Dijon and Honey with Lemon Juice
Unilever Best Foods
800-9-lawrys www.lawrys.com
Bottom Line: 20 calories per serving (1 tbsp)
Details: Yummy Hunters say it's a great complement to chicken breasts. They add they like to pour it onto baked potatoes. *Helen:* A great marinade for fish and a must marinade for mustard lovers. *Eric:* Like Romeo and Juliet, like Antony and Cleopatra—Dijon and Honey. A combo for the ages.
Availability: Supermarkets and online

✳ Dill Mustard
The Silver Palate, Dill Mustard Grilling Sauce
The Silver Palate
201-568-0110 www.silverpalate.com
Bottom Line: 80 calories per serving (2 tbsp)
Details: Yummy Hunters rave about the dill — mustard combo and tell us it livens up all the chicken meals they find themselves eating. *Helen & Eric:* We put it on a piece of salmon and the combination of flavors was wonderfully delicious.
Availability: Supermarkets, by phone at 866-927-6879 and online

✱ Garlic & Rosemary
Stone Wall Kitchen, Garlic & Rosemary Citrus Sauce
Stone Wall Kitchen
800-207-5267 www.stonewallkitchen.com
Bottom Line: 40 calories per serving (2 tbsp)
Details: Yummy Hunters told us they used it to cook a piece of fillet of sole and this dish tasted like something out of a gourmet restaurant. *Helen:* My daughter just followed our Yummy Hunters' suggestion and prepared the most fabulous lunch I've had in weeks. This is one special-tasting marinade. *Eric:* Another great meal I missed. Thanks a lot!
Availability: Supermarkets and online

✱ Honey Smoke
KC Masterpiece, Honey Smoke, Steak Sauce
The HV Food Products Company
800-537-2823 www.kcmasterpiece.com
Bottom Line: 50 calories per serving (2 tbsp)
Details: Yummy Hunters who need their meat tell us this is their favorite barbecue sauce. They add a steak just isn't a steak unless they use KC Masterpiece steak sauce. *Helen:* Oh, this is really good! *Eric:* While Helen's totally overcome by rapture, let me say we had it on chicken and it gave it a mouth-watering backyard-barbecue flavor.
Availability: Supermarkets and club stores

✱ Mesquite with Lime Juice
Lawry's, 30 Minute Marinade Mesquite with Lime Juice
Unilever Best Foods
800-9-lawrys www.lawrys.com
Bottom Line: 5 calories per serving (1 tbsp)
Details: Yummy Hunters enjoy the smoky flavor and love it on chicken and burgers. *Helen:* Lime juice adds a refreshing tartness to this authentic mesquite marinade. We spread it on turkey burgers, turning them into a taste sensation. *Eric:* I'm always amazed at how a marinade can transform the ordinary into the extraordinary.
Availability: Supermarkets and online

* Steak House
Peter Luger, Steak House Old Fashioned Steak Sauce
Peter Luger Enterprises, Inc.
718-387-0500 www.peterluger.com
Bottom Line: 30 calories per serving (1 tbsp)
Details: Yummy Hunters use it on steaks and as a marinade for chicken. *Helen:* We followed the company's serving suggestions from the website, mixing low-fat mayo with the sauce, and made the best Russian dressing we ever had. *Eric:* This will have to hold me until I make it to Peter Luger's.
Availability: Supermarkets in New York, New Jersey, Florida, by phone and online

* Veri Veri Teriyaki
Soy Vay, Veri Veri Teriyaki
Soy Vay
800-600-2077 www.soyvay.com
Bottom Line: 35 calories per serving (1 tbsp)
Details: Yummy Hunters rave this is no ordinary teriyaki sauce. They swear it's the sesame seeds that set this sauce apart from the rest. *Helen:* Maybe it is the sesame seeds, or maybe it's because it's so thick. This is unlike any teriyaki sauce we've ever tried. We think it's just the perfect combination of oriental flavorings. We marinated a piece of swordfish for a few hours and then barbecued it. Scrumptious! *Eric:* Veri Veri Teriyaki is very, very good. Soy vay!
Availability: Supermarkets and online

* Worcestershire for Chicken
Lea & Perrins, Worcestershire for Chicken
Lea & Perrins
800-987-4674 www.leaperrins.com
Bottom Line: 0 calories per serving (1 tsp)
Details: Yummy Hunters say this sauce is the perfect complement when cooking poultry. Some like to use it as a marinade, whereas others pour it over cooked chicken. *Helen:* We tried it over a piece of cooked chicken. It made the chicken come alive with flavor! *Eric:* Lip-smacking good!
Availability: Supermarkets

OILS

✳ Olive

Spectrum Naturals, Extra Virgin Olive, Spray Oil
Spectrum Organic Products, Inc.
800-995-2705 www.spectrumorganics.com
Bottom Line: 0 calories per serving (⅓ second spray)
Details: Yummy Hunters like this easy spray container and say that for cooking things from eggs to vegetables it makes the foods just as tasty as using butter, yet doesn't add unwanted calories. *Helen:* Although I feel olive oil adds a much nicer flavor than butter, I still want you to understand that even though the container says 0 calories, that is only for a third of a second's worth of spray. *Eric:* Partner, don't get trigger happy.
Availability: Supermarkets

✳ Olive Oil

Pam, Cooking Spray, Olive Oil
International Home Foods, Inc.
800-726-4908 www.pam4you.com
Bottom Line: 0 calories per serving (⅓ second spray)
Details: Yummy Hunters exclaim it's a great cooking spray and they use it when sautéing. *Helen & Eric:* Be warned—who sprays for that length of time? We also use the Butter flavor and it's equally good.
Availability: Supermarkets

SEASONINGS

✳ Cajun

Kernel Season's, Cajun, Popcorn Seasoning
Kernel Season's LLC
773-292-4567 www.nomorenakedpopcorn.com
Bottom Line: 2 calories per serving (¼ tsp)
Details: Yummy Hunters who love Cajun food enjoy putting this on boiled shrimp and pretzels. *Helen & Eric:* This is some great brand and the product uses are endless. Other tantalizing flavors at 2 calories are Parmesan & Garlic and White Cheddar.
Availability: Online

✳ Garden Vegetable
McCormick, Salad Toppins, Garden Vegetable
McCormick & Co. Inc.
800-632-5847 www.mccormick.com
Bottom Line: 35 calories per serving (1⅓ tbsp)
Details: Yummy Hunters say it adds extra flavor to a basic salad. *Helen:* It's got everything you might want—carrots, onions, red peppers, sunflower seeds and more. Crunchy, unique and so so easy. *Eric:* All you've got to do is shake straight from the bottle and you've got a crunchy, gourmet salad.
Availability: Supermarkets

✳ Garlic Herb
McCormick 1 Step Garlic Herb for Chicken
McCormick & Co., Inc.
800-632-5847 www.mccormick.com
Bottom Line: 15 calories per serving (¾ tsp)
Details: Yummy Hunters say when they're dieting, they find themselves eating a lot of chicken, so naturally they're always looking for ways to spice it up. This product does the trick. *Helen:* We sprinkled this on a chicken breast and then broiled. Yummy! *Eric:* It has just the right amount of garlic and seasoning in an easy-to-use shaker. For some, like me, who are "seasoning challenged," it made me into a seasoned expert.
Availability: Supermarkets

✳ Peanut
A Taste of Thai, Spicy Thai Peanut Bake
Andre Prost, Inc.
800-243-0897 www.atasteofthai.com
Bottom Line: 45 calories per serving (¼ envelope)
Details: Yummy Hunters say this is a really easy meal. All they have to do is dip chicken in fat-free milk, put it in a bag with this peanut sauce, shake and bake. One adds her family, who ordinarily don't like exotic or ethnic foods, ate it up. *Helen:* I'm so pleased that Thai food has found its way into the diet world. This seasoning is a taste sensation. *Eric:* Thai me up, Thai me down. This really Thai-ed me over.

Availability: Supermarkets, health food stores; store locations and ordering online

✱ Romano Cheese

McCormick, Salad Supreme Seasoning, Romano Cheese

McCormick & Co., Inc.

800-632-5847 www.mccormick.com

Bottom Line: 15 calories per serving (¼ tsp)

Details: Yummy Hunters use this on cold pasta— and it's so good. *Helen & Eric:* It tastes like a cross between celery and paprika. Try it on a cold cucumber salad.

Availability: Supermarkets

✱ Sweet Onion & Pepper

McCormick 1 Step, Sweet Onion & Pepper

McCormick & Co., Inc.

800-632-5847 www.mccormick.com

Bottom Line: 15 calories per serving (½ tsp)

Details: Some Yummy Hunters stew a big pot of veggies so when they're hungry they can scoop out a bowl. Nothing makes this dish work better than Sweet Onion & Pepper seasoning. *Helen & Eric:* Tasty good with a real kick, so use it sparingly.

Availability: Supermarkets

SPICES

✱ Mesquite

Mrs. Dash, Grilling Blends, Mesquite

Alberto-Culver, USA, Inc.

800-622-3274 www.mrsdash.com

Bottom Line: 0 calories (¼ tsp)

Details: One Yummy Hunter, on her doctors' advice, watched her salt intake. After a sea of bland and flavorless products, she discovered this thrilling spice. *Helen & Eric:* We didn't miss the salt at all. We used it to broil a piece of swordfish, and it added a delicious mesquite flavor. Also comes in these Yummy flavors: Original, Garlic & Herb, Extra Spicy, Lemon Pepper and Tomato Basil Garlic.

Availability: Supermarkets

SWEETENERS

✱ Artificial Sweetener
Splenda, Artificial Sweetener
Splenda Division of McNeil-PPC, Inc.
800-777-5363 www.splenda.com
Bottom Line: 0 calories per serving (1 packet)
Details: Yummy Hunters used the pink package, then the blue and now they're yellow, through and through. *Helen & Eric:* The number one choice of Yummy Hunters, especially those on low-carb diets.
Availability: Supermarkets, health food stores and ordering online at www.netgrocer.com

✱ Natural Sweetener
Sweet Leaf, Stevia Plus, Natural Sweetener
Wisdom Herbs
800-899-9908 www.wisdomnaturalbrands.com
Bottom Line: 0 calories per serving (½ packet)
Details: Yummy Hunters like this better than the artificial brands. It makes everything taste sweeter. *Helen & Eric:* A little goes a long way. The choice when you want more of a natural product.
Availability: Supermarkets and health food stores

✱ Sugar
Hain Pure Foods, Organic Sugar
Hain Celestial Group, Inc.
800-434-4246 www.hain-celestial.com
Bottom Line: 10 calories per serving (1 tbsp)
Details: Yummy Hunters who don't like using artificial sweeteners enjoy using this 10-calorie option. *Helen:* Beware, this is real sugar. Ten calories did not sweeten my coffee—needed 30. *Eric:* You are my sugar girl, you got me wanting you.
Availability: Supermarkets, health food stores and ordering online at www.naturemart.com

The older you get, the tougher it is to lose weight, because by then your body and your fat are really good friends.

SIDES
COUSCOUS, PASTA, POLENTA,
RICE, VEGETABLES

M‍Y MOM tried to get me to eat vegetables; Eric's
warned him against sipping his spaghetti. I'm
still in a love—hate relationship with veggies 'cause
I'd rather have a cookie than a carrot stick. Eric
still would be sucking up his noodles if he didn't
have to suck in his stomach afterward. Thanks to
our Yummy Hunters, there is hope for us both.

COUSCOUS

✻ Nutted with Currants & Spice
Casbah, Couscous, Nutted with Currants & Spice
Hain Celestial Group, Inc.
800-434-4246 www.casbahnaturalfoods.com
Bottom Line: 160 calories per serving (¼ cup dry)
Details: Yummy Hunters make this at night and
bring it into the office the next day cold. It's so
filling and satisfying. *Helen & Eric:* A unique flavor
that makes the perfect side for any main meal.
Availability: Supermarkets

PASTA

Egg Fettuccini
**Al Dente, Carba-Nada, Reduced Carb Pasta, Egg
Fettuccini**
Al Dente, Inc.
734-449-8522 www.aldentepasta.com
Bottom Line: 140 calories per serving (2 oz)
Details: Yummy Hunters say they found their thrill
in this low-carb pasta. One adds she switched to
this pasta and her family had no idea she'd made
any change. *Helen & Eric:* The rich flavor of this
pasta will win over low-carb and low-cal dieters
alike. This won't disappoint!
Availability: Supermarkets and online

Get the latest info at **www.yummyhunters.com**   245

Penne Rigate
Ronzoni, Healthy Harvest, Whole Wheat Blend Pasta
New World Pasta Co.
800-730-5957 www.healthyharvestpasta.com
Bottom Line: 180 calories per serving (2 oz)
Details: Yummy Hunters who don't enjoy low-carb diets tell us they can still get their fill of pasta with this full-flavored whole wheat side. Another says this delicious pasta helped her stay on her diet and maintain her 20-pound weight loss. *Helen & Eric:* We steamed vegetables and added it to this pasta with a little olive oil and garlic.
Availability: Supermarkets and wholesale clubs

* Spinach/Whole Wheat
Hodgson Mill, Whole Wheat Spinach Spaghetti
Hodgson Mill, Inc.
800-525-0177 www.hodgsonmill.com
Bottom Line: 190 calories prepared (2 oz dry)
Details: Yummy Hunters who normally have to avoid pasta when dieting tell us this tasty, high-fiber spaghetti is a real treat. *Helen:* Interesting taste. Try it with steamed spinach, garlic and a little olive oil on top. *Eric:* Rich taste. Not too chewy. Very different and very good.
Availability: Some supermarkets, by phone and online

* Tofu Shirataki
House, Tofu Shirataki
House Foods America Corporation
714-901-4350 www.house-foods.com
Bottom Line: 20 calories per serving (4 oz)
Details: *Helen:* I found this at a local heath food store, and I'm bursting with excitement. This ingenious product looks and tastes just like spaghetti even though it's tofu! I tried it with my favorite tomato sauce and also dropped it into a pot of chicken soup. *Eric:* Not only is it as good as spaghetti, but *tofu* is much easier to spell.
Availability: Supermarkets, health food stores and ordering online at www.gethealthyamerica.com

POLENTA

Original
Nate's, Organic Polenta, Original
Monterey Pasta Company
800-588-7782 www.montereypasta.com
Bottom Line: 80 calories per serving (4 oz)
Details: Yummy Hunters who grew up eating starches (polenta being one of them) tell us they started to read labels when their waistline started expanding. They are surprised their favorite polenta is only 80 calories. *Helen & Eric:* We loved the consistency and the super corn flavor.
Availability: Supermarkets and health food stores; store locations online

RICE

✳ Rice and Red Beans
Goya, Rice and Red Beans
Goya Foods, Inc.
201-348-4900 www.goya.com
Bottom Line: 160 calories per serving (¼ cup)
Details: Yummy Hunters say it's great to get away from meat and chicken, and this supplies variety to their dieting menu needs. *Helen & Eric:* We found we needed a triple serving to make it a satisfying meal. At a 160 calories, it makes for a great side dish. Add a little salsa for some extra fun.
Availability: Supermarkets and ordering online at www.netgrocer.com

Thai Coconut Ginger
Lundberg, Rice Sensations, Thai Coconut Ginger
Lundberg Family Farms
530-882-4551 www.lundberg.com
Bottom Line: 114 calories per serving (½ cup)
Details: Yummy Hunters say this is no boring rice dish. Half a cup on the side of a piece of chicken does the trick. *Helen & Eric:* The coconut ginger combo is uniquely delicious.
Availability: Supermarkets, health food stores and ordering online at www.leesmarket.com

* Wild Rice
Lundberg, Wild Blend, Gourmet Wild & Brown Rices
Lundberg Family Farms
530-882-4551 www.lundberg.com
Bottom Line: 150 calories per serving (¼ cup)
Details: Yummy Hunters declare they love the blending of rices. They sauté onions and Olive Oil Pam and then add that to the rice and it's really terrific. *Helen & Eric:* A great consistency that we thought needed a little flavor, so we added chicken broth. What a wonderful dish it was.
Availability: Supermarkets, health food stores and ordering online at www.leesmarket.com

VEGETABLES

Bean, Baked
Amy's Organic Vegetarian Beans
Amy's Kitchen
707-578-7188 www.amyskitchen.com
Bottom Line: 120 calories per serving (½ cup)
Details: Yummy Hunters who love hot dogs tell us they have finally found the perfect complement, thanks to this baked bean delight from Amy's. *Helen & Eric:* Terrific, slightly sweet with a savory tomato flavor. We loved them beans!
Availability: Health food stores, supermarkets and some club stores; store locations online

* Black Beans, Refried
Amy's Vegetarian Organic Refried Beans
Amy's Kitchen
707-578-7188 www.amyskitchen.com
Bottom Line: 140 calories per serving (½ cup)
Details: One Yummy Hunter says she sprinkles a handful of shredded light cheese on top, mics it for 2 – 3 minutes on high, then serves it with baked tortilla chips and really wows her guests! *Helen & Eric:* We put these beans in a soft tortilla and added a few grilled chicken strips. Yum, yum.
Availability: Health food stores, supermarkets and some club stores; store locations online

* Chop Suey Vegetables
La Choy, Chop Suey Vegetables
ConAgra Foods, Inc.
800-338-8831 www.conagrafoods.com
Bottom Line: 15 calories per serving (½ cup)
Details: Yummy Hunters say when dieting they get both physically and emotionally hungry, and this delicious chop suey with vegetables has a great Chinese taste and its crunchiness is satisfying. *Helen:* Half a cup of this will get you through any sort of hunger crisis. Always keep a can on hand. *Eric:* How do you say *amen* in Chinese?
Availability: Supermarkets

* Early Peas
Le Sueur, Very Young Small Early Peas
General Mills, Inc.
800-998-9996 www.pillsbury.com
Bottom Line: 60 calories per serving (½ cup)
Details: Yummy Hunters confess when they're on a diet, the best way to curb their appetite is to heat up a can of these sweet and delicious peas and eat them right out of the saucepan. *Helen & Eric:* These baby peas are tender and delicious. For variety, try sprinkling a little veggie Parmesan on top.
Availability: Supermarkets

* Potato, French Fries
Nathan's Jumbo Crinkle Cut French Fries
ConAgra Foods, Inc.
800-338-8831 www.conagrafoods.com
Bottom Line: 110 calories per serving (14 pieces)
Details: One Yummy Hunter was thrilled to discover this childhood favorite in her local supermarket and is excited to see thes fries could fit into her diet plan. Yummy Hunters who know the name Nathan's are overjoyed to discover they can now eat this famous brand's delicious french fries. *Helen:* Big, potatoey and delicious. Boy, do these bring back some great memories. *Eric:* For me too! I can even remember the smell of the salt sea air at Coney Island.
Availability: Supermarkets and online

Potato, Sweet
Alexia, Sweet Potato, Hanna Gold Julienne Fries with Sea Salt
Alexia Foods
718-609-5665 www.alexiafoods.com
Bottom Line: 140 calories per serving (24 pieces)
Details: Yummy Hunters who love sweet potatoes tell us these delicious fries take sweet potato taste to new heights. *Helen:* I love sweet potatoes so this is a real treat for me. *Eric:* They set the gold standard in fries.
Availability: Supermarkets and health food stores

Potatoes, Mashed
Barbara's, Mashed Potatoes
Barbara's For A Brighter Future
707-765-2273 www.barbarasbakery.com
Bottom Line: 70 calories per serving (½ cup prepared)
Details: When Yummy Hunters want an easy side dish they say Barbara's cooks up light and fluffy and tastes delicious. *Helen:* Who doesn't like mashed potatoes? *Eric:* You're going to shovel this creamy dish down without coming up for air.
Availability: Health food stores and some supermarkets; store locations online

Squash, Winter
Cascadian Farm, Winter Squash
General Mills, Inc.
800-624-4123 www.cfarm.com
Bottom Line: 70 calories per serving (½ cup)
Details: Yummy Hunters say this is the perfect side. It's creamy like mashed potatoes yet filling and low in calories. *Helen:* For between-meal hunger try a bowl of this squash. *Eric:* So good it should be named "All-Year-Round Squash."
Availability: Supermarkets and health food stores; store locations online

He who takes medicine and neglects diet wastes the skill of the physician.
—Chinese Proverb

✱ A Low-Fat Product

SOUPS

Soup's on! What two words can convey more emotions or evoke more memories? Our Yummy Hunters couldn't agree more and have discovered a delicious array of soups that will cure whatever ails you.

✳ Black Bean
Walnut Acres, Organic, Hearty Black Bean
Hain Celestial Group, Inc.
866-492-5688 www.walnutacres.com
Bottom Line: 150 calories per serving (1 cup)
Details: Yummy Hunters tell us when they want a warm, filling and delicious soup this is their favorite choice. *Helen:* Great-tasting soup. Tender beans, a light touch of corn. It's delish. *Eric:* So hearty with flavor and goodness, you'll be singing pirate songs and calling everyone matey!
Availability: Supermarkets

✳ Cabbage Soup
Tabatchnick, Cabbage Soup
Tabatchnick Fine Food, Inc.
732-247-6668 www.tabatchnick.com
Bottom Line: 60 calories per serving (1 pouch)
Details: Yummy Hunters say this soup is very sweet tasting and it tides them over between meals. *Helen:* Tasted like the cabbage soup my grandma used to make. *Eric:* I wasn't as fortunate, so I'm making up for a lost childhood.
Availability: Frozen kosher section of supermarkets and online

✳ Cha-Cha
Fantastic, Cha-Cha Chili, Big Soup Cup
Fantastic Foods, Inc.
800-288-1089 www.fantasticfoods.com
Bottom Line: 220 calories per serving (62 g)
Details: Yummy Hunters who don't eat meat love this veggie delight. They rave about the flavor and the convenience. *Helen:* Full chili taste in a big bowl of soup. The container we tried held two servings and not only did it taste great but filled us up, too. *Eric:* I never had chili soup before. Hot-cha-cha!
Availability: Supermarkets, health food stores and club stores; store locations and ordering online and at www.leesmarket.com

✳ Chicken
Herb Ox, Chicken Bullion
Hormel Foods Corp.
800-523-4635 www.hormel.com
Bottom Line: 5 calories per serving (1 cube)
Details: Yummy Hunters use this instead of butter on mashed potatoes and save a ton of calories. *Helen:* We carved out the top of a whole onion, put one cube in with a little water, then covered and microwaved until tender. We also gave brown rice a fabulous chicken flavor by adding two cubes to the water. *Eric:* Don't forget to have a hankie close by when you peel the onion. Also available in beef.
Availability: Supermarkets and online

✳ Chicken
Imagine, Organic, Free Range, Chicken Broth
Hain Celestial Group, Inc.
800-434-4246 www.imaginefoods.com
Bottom Line: 20 calories per serving (1 cup)
Details: Yummy Hunters use this chicken broth to cook a pot of vegetables and say that it adds flavor without calories. *Helen:* Try taking a baked potato, mashing it up and using this broth instead of butter for a delicious low-cal side dish. *Eric:* Good for what ails ya!
Availability: Health food stores

* Chicken Creamy Broccoli
Imagine, Creamy Broccoli Soup
Hain Celestial Group, Inc.
800-434-4246 www.imaginefoods.com
Bottom Line: 70 calories per serving (1 cup)
Details: Yummy Hunters rave this is their all-time favorite cream soup and they cannot get enough of its goodness. One Yummy Hunter who can't get enough broccoli added fresh broccoli and a few carrots and told us it was delish. *Helen:* I took this soup and mixed it with Barbara's Mashed Potato and created a great side sensation. *Eric:* One creamy delicious dish. Next time I'm going to try our Yummy Hunter's recipe.
Availability: Health food stores

* Chicken Noodle
Campbell's, Classics, Homestyle, Chicken Noodle
Campbell Soup Company
800-257-8443 www.campbellsoup.com
Bottom Line: 70 calories per serving (½ cup)
Details: Yummy Hunters say it tastes just like Mom's chicken soup. *Helen:* This classic chicken soup is loaded with tender noodles and reminds me of the soup my grandmother made. *Eric:* Few products can be called classic. This one is classic in every sense of the word.
Availability: Supermarkets and ordering online at www.netgrocer.com

* Chicken Noodle
Walnut Acres, Homestyle, Organic Chicken Noodle
Hain Celestial Group, Inc.
866-492-5688 www.walnutacres.com
Bottom Line: 80 calories per serving (1 cup)
Details: Yummy Hunters tell us this is as good as the soup they had growing up as kids. They love the homestyle taste of this chicken noodle soup. *Helen:* Tender broad noodles add a special flair to this homestyle favorite. *Eric:* Cluck, cluck! This will have you "doing the Chicken Dance".
Availability: Supermarkets

✱ Corn & Potato Chowder
Fantastic, Corn & Potato Chowder, Big Soup Cup
Fantastic Foods, Inc.
800-288-1089 www.fantasticfoods.com
Bottom Line: 130 calories per serving (36 g)
Details: Yummy Hunters tell us they tried it because it sounded interesting and they weren't disappointed. They said the corn and potatoes make a very nice combination. *Helen:* Sweet corn blended with perfect, tasty white potatoes. *Eric:* I love corn chowder and this one is rich and hearty and extremely filling.
Availability: Supermarkets, health food stores and club stores; store locations and ordering online and at www.leesmarket.com

Cream of Broccoli
Campbell's, Soup at Hand, Cream of Broccoli
Campbell Soup Company
800-257-8443 www.campbellsoup.com
Bottom Line: 150 calories per serving (10¾ oz)
Details: Yummy Hunters say when they're dieting, they like foods that taste like the real thing. The calorie count of this soup attracted them, but the creamy taste of broccoli kept them coming back. *Helen:* If you like cream of broccoli, you'll love this rich-tasting soup. We each had one can for lunch and with a few crackers it was satisfyingly filling. *Eric:* Overwhelmingly good. It's the crème de la cream of broccoli soup.
Availability: Supermarkets

✱ Creamy Potato with Broccoli
Health Valley, Fat-Free, Creamy Potato with Broccoli Soup
Hain Celestial Group, Inc.
800-423-4846 www.hain-celestial.com
Bottom Line: 80 calories per serving (⅓ cup)
Details: Yummy Hunters say this is a delicious, low-cal way to eat one of their favorite foods. *Helen & Eric:* If you're a potato lover (and who's not), this soup is a must!
Availability: Supermarkets and health food stores

SOUPS

✳ Egg Drop
Croyden House, Egg Drop Soup Mix
Rokeach Food Distributors, Inc.
973-491-9696 www.rokeach.com
Bottom Line: 30 calories per serving (1 tbsp)
Details: One Yummy Hunter tells us she and her husband share a bowl every Thursday evening and follow it with a sweet and sour entrée and call it their "Chinese Night Out." *Helen & Eric:* We have always loved egg drop soup and this is the first store-bought brand that live up to the original.
Availability: Supermarkets

✳ Escarole in Chicken Broth
Progresso, Classics Soup, Escarole in Chicken Broth
General Mills, Inc.
800-200-9377 www.progressosoup.com
Bottom Line: 25 calories per serving (1 cup)
Details: Yummy Hunters are saying it warms and fills them up for a small amount of calories. They declare they have been eating this soup for years and just love it, especially when they cut up tofu and throw it in while the soup is heating. *Helen & Eric:* When it's cold outside, just pop open a can of this soup, and it's great for in between meals.
Availability: Supermarkets and ordering online at www.netgrocer.com

✳ Garlic Herb
Fantastic, Garlic Herb, Recipe Mix Soup & Dip
Fantastic Foods, Inc.
800-288-1089 www.fantasticfoods.com
Bottom Line: 20 calories per serving (1 cup prepared)
Details: Yummy Hunters recommend mixing this soup with fat-free sour cream and then eating it with baked potato chips. One suggests sprinkling a little on a chicken cutlet before you bake it. *Helen:* We made soup using half the amount of water and tons of fresh veggies. Marvelous! *Eric:* This soup was subtly delicious and a real gourmet treat.
Availability: Supermarkets, health food stores and club stores; store locations and ordering online

* Lentil
Progresso, Lentil Soup
General Mills, Inc.
800-200-9377 www.progressosoup.com
Bottom Line: 130 calories per serving (1 cup)
Details: One Yummy Hunter tells us that her two-year-old would eat only this soup for lunch. One day the Yummy Hunter tried a spoonful and realized her child was onto something. She adds that it's one of the new foods she's been eating that has helped her lose 30 pounds. *Helen:* These appetizing lentils make for a very filling soup. *Eric:* Hearty har har!
Availability: Supermarkets

* Manhattan Clam Chowder
Progresso, Manhattan Clam Chowder
General Mills, Inc.
800-200-9377 www.progressosoup.com
Bottom Line: 110 calories per serving (1 cup)
Details: Our Yummy Hunters rave about the chunky, juicy clams. Another dieter, who grew up eating clam chowder, says that now, thanks to Progresso, she can eat a tasty clam chowder that fits with her diet. *Helen:* We love the great-tasting tomato base. *Eric:* Fresh clam taste in a classic chowder. Delicious!
Availability: Supermarkets and ordering online at www.netgrocer.com

* Minestrone
Progresso, Minestrone Soup
General Mills, Inc.
800-200-9377 www.progressosoup.com
Bottom Line: 110 calories per serving (1 cup)
Details: One Yummy Hunter says she doesn't like soup out of a can, but when she recently started a diet, she tried this soup and discovered it not only tastes homemade but fits into her plan. *Helen & Eric:* We split the can and a grilled cheese sandwich (made with a butter substitute, of course), and it was a wonderfully satisfying meal.
Availability: Supermarkets

✳ Miso
Imagine, California Miso, Organic Broth
Hain Celestial Group, Inc.
800-434-4246 www.imaginefoods.com
Bottom Line: 30 calories per serving (1 cup)
Details: Yummy Hunters say they always order Miso soup when they go to a Japanese restaurant and they are overjoyed to discover this authentic-tasting, low-cal, low-fat version. *Helen:* I added tofu for an even more filling meal. For exotic results when cooking rice, substitute this soup for water and you're in for a real treat. *Eric:* Sounds delicious. When do I get an invite?
Availability: Supermarkets and health food stores

✳ Onion
Tabatchnick, Frenchman's Onion Soup
Tabatchnick Fine Food, Inc.
732-247-6668 www.tabatchnick.com
Bottom Line: 50 calories per serving (1 pouch)
Details: Yummy Hunters tell us this soup is every bit as good as they get in a French bistro. They say it's appetizing and satisfying. *Helen:* Be careful vegetarians, this soup is made with beef broth. *Eric:* When I think of a French bistro, I melt a little light mozzarella and make it au gratin!
Availability: Frozen kosher section of most supermarkets and online

✳ Pizza
Campbell's, Soup At Hand, Pizza
Campbell Soup Company
800-257-8443 www.campbellsoup.com
Bottom Line: 140 calories per serving (10¾ oz)
Details: Yummy Hunters say it's pizza on the go and wonder what Campbell will think of next. They add that getting full for 130 calories is a real treat. *Helen:* Although it didn't taste like pizza to us, it had a very appealing smoky flavor. *Eric:* No, we didn't overcook it!
Availability: Supermarkets and ordering online at www.netgrocer.com

✱ Split Pea
Amy's, Organic Soups, Low Fat, Split Pea
Amy's Kitchen, Inc.
707-578-7188 www.amyskitchen.com
Bottom Line: 100 calories per serving (1 cup)
Details: Yummy Hunters tell us how richly authentic this soup is. *Helen:* As a kid I hated peas but loved tomatoes, so my grandmother called pea soup green tomato soup. This is the best "green tomato" soup I've ever had. *Eric:* Whatever you call it, this is delicious.
Availability: Health food stores, supermarkets and some club stores; store locations online and ordering at www.nomeat.com

✱ Split Pea
Streits, Split Pea Soup Mix
Aron Streits, Inc.
212-475-7000 www.streitsmatzos.com
Bottom Line: 144 calories per serving (1 cup prepared)
Details: Yummy Hunters name this their favorite comfort soup. They loved the aroma, the taste and the general good feelings associated with it. *Helen:* While preparing this soup, the aroma made our mouths water. *Eric:* Beware, using this soup as a room freshener will just invite all your neighbors in for a meal!
Availability: Supermarkets and ordering online at www.groceryfinder.com and www.netgrocer.com

✱ Split Pea & Carrots
Health Valley, Split Pea & Carrots Soup
Hain Celestial Group, Inc.
800-423-4846 www.hain-celestial.com
Bottom Line: 110 calories per serving (1 cup)
Details: Yummy Hunters love the great taste and the fact this soup has no fat or cholesterol. Easy to grab when they're hungry. *Helen & Eric:* Thick and hearty pea soup loaded with tender carrots makes this classic soup even more memorable.
Availability: Supermarkets, health food stores and ordering online at www.naturemart.com

∗ Tofu Miso
Kikkoman, Tofu Miso Soup
Kikkoman, Int'l, Inc.
www.kikkoman.com
Bottom Line: 30 calories per serving (1 packet)
Details: Yummy Hunters say this soup is delicious, curbs their appetite and they never leave a drop left over. *Helen & Eric:* Another Japanese favorite that lives up to the original.
Availability: Supermarkets

∗ Tomato
Campbell's, Soup at Hand, Classic Tomato
Campbell Soup Company
800-257-8443 www.campbellsoup.com
Bottom Line: 120 calories per serving (10¾-oz container)
Details: Yummy Hunters say Campbell's is still their favorite tomato soup and they love the fact they can now take this handy portion-controlled container with them to work. They add it fills them up and helps keep them on their diet. *Helen:* Campbell's always has, and continues to make, the best tomato soup I've ever eaten. *Eric:* Umm, umm, good.
Availability: Supermarkets and ordering online at www.netgrocer.com

∗ Vegetable
Health Valley, Fat-Free, Vegetable Broth
Hain Celestial Group, Inc.
800-423-4846 www.hain-celestial.com
Bottom Line: 20 calories per serving (1 cup)
Details: Yummy Hunters eat it plain on a winter's day. They also like to use it as a base for vegetable soup and in recipes. *Helen:* It has a garden-fresh flavor that enhances any recipe. *Eric:* We agree with our Yummy Hunters that it's robust enough to stand on its own, with, of course, the addition of some low-fat croutons.
Availability: Supermarkets, health food stores, and ordering online at www.leesmarket.com, www.naturemart.com and www.netgrocer.com

✳ White Bean
Alessi, Traditional Tuscan, White Bean Soup
Vigo Importing Co., Inc.
www.vigoalessi.com
Bottom Line: 150 calories per serving (1 cup prepared)
Details: Yummy Hunters enjoy preparing this restaurant-quality soup. *Helen & Eric:* The tender white bean and the special spices make for a very remarkable-tasting soup.
Availability: Supermarkets and ordering online and at www.netgrocer.com

✳ White Bean
Walnut Acres, Organic, Tuscan White Bean
Hain Celestial Group, Inc.
866-492-5688 www.walnutacres.com
Bottom Line: 130 calories per serving (1 cup)
Details: One Yummy Hunter, who normally likes to make all her soups from scratch, traded that job in for the homemade taste of this soup. *Helen:* Mediterranean-inspired soup is sure to be a palate pleaser. *Eric:* Best-tasting bean soup under the Tuscan sun.
Availability: Supermarkets

I just ate my willpower.

SPREADS

BUTTER, CREAM CHEESE, JAMS/JELLIES,
PEANUT BUTTER, TOMATO, YOGURT SPREADS

W E'RE SPREADING THE NEWS that these tasty
products will add flavor to your foods without
adding an excessive amount of calories.

————

BUTTER

* Apple Butter
Eden Foods, Inc.
Spectrum Organic Products, Inc.
888-441-3336 www.edenfoods.com
Bottom Line: 20 calories per serving (1 tbps)
Details: Yummy Hunters say this is really good
stuff. They say it makes any piece of toast or bread
a sweet treat. *Helen & Eric:* Wow! Jelly, move aside.
Availability: Health food stores

* Buttery
Smart Balance, Light, Buttery Spread
GFA Brands, Inc.
201-568-9300 www.smartbalance.com
Bottom Line: 45 calories per serving (1 tbsp)
Details: Yummy Hunters say besides loving the
taste, it has no hydrogenated fat, so it makes
their doctors very happy. *Helen:* We tried it on
bread, crackers, even made eggs with it and it
tastes and spreads like butter to us. *Eric:* Oh, the
marvels of modern science!
Availability: Supermarkets

CREAM CHEESE

Cream Cheese
Tofutti, Cream Cheese, Better Than Cream Cheese
Tofutti Brands, Inc.
908-272-2400 www.tofutti.com
Bottom Line: 80 calories per serving (1 oz)
Details: Senior citizens inform us that cheese products upset their stomachs, so when a nurse told a Yummy Hunter about this cheese, she tried it and loved it. *Helen & Eric:* A terrific, cheesy taste. If we hadn't spooned it out ourselves, we would have never known the difference.
Availability: Supermarkets and health food stores

JAMS/JELLIES

* Amaretto Apricot
Country Cupboard, Amaretto Apricot
Country Cupboard
800-382-3267 www.countrycupboard.com
Bottom Line: 5 calories per serving (1 tbsp)
Details: *Helen:* We couldn't believe our luck when we sampled this delicious spread that goes great with a little butter spray or just by itself on some whole wheat bread. *Eric:* What a great combo—makes for a uniquely delicious and exotically different treat.
Availability: Online

* Boysenberry
Polaner, All Fruit, Boysenberry
B&G Foods, Inc.
www.allfruit.com
Bottom Line: 40 calories per serving (1 tbsp)
Details: Yummy Hunters put this spread on their English muffins and the delicious taste gives them a great start to a day of dieting. *Helen:* A happy breakfast keeps you motivated all day. *Eric:* We spread some on buckwheat pancakes and what a sweet treat.
Availability: Supermarkets and ordering online at www.mybrands.com

* A Low-Fat Product

* Orange
Smuckers, Orange Light Sugar Free Marmalade
J.M. Smuckers

888-550-9555 www.smuckers.com

Bottom Line: 10 calories per serving (1 tbsp)

Details: Yummy Hunters mix this with cottage cheese in the morning and say it adds a sweet, citrus flavor. *Helen:* If you love orange marmalade, spread this on anything and everything. We particularly love the chewy, tasty orange rinds. *Eric:* Warning: This can be dangerous when licked off a sharp knife. Use only with an oversized spoon.

Availability: Supermarkets and online

* Peach
Shiloh Farms, All Natural Peach Spread
Shiloh Farms

800-362-6832 users.nwark.com/~shilohf

Bottom Line: 30 calories per serving (1 tbsp)

Details: One Yummy Hunter relates that she first tried this spread over a year ago at a spa. She brought a jar home and has been ordering it ever since. *Helen:* You can really taste the natural, homemade flavor. This product doesn't have any artificial sweeteners, so the calories are a little higher — but rest assured, a little goes a long way. *Eric:* Brimming with natural peachy goodness. Sweeter than sweet. A peach of a peach.

Availability: By phone

* Red Raspberry
Smuckers, Light Sugar Free Red Raspberry Preserves
J.M. Smuckers

888-550-9555 www.smuckers.com

Bottom Line: 10 calories per serving (1 tbsp)

Details: Our Yummy Hunters confess they are very boring and eat the same breakfast every morning: whole wheat toast with Smuckers Red Raspberry Preserves. They say it keeps them eating right all day. *Helen & Eric:* Our Yummy Hunters have it right; however, we jazzed it up a bit by adding some Smart Balance Buttery Spread.

Availability: Supermarkets and online

✱ Wild Forest Berry
Country Cupboard, Wild Forest Berry Preserves
Country Cupboard
800-382-3267 www.countrycupboard.com
Bottom Line: 5 calories per serving (1 tbsp)
Details: Yummy Hunters cannot believe this sweet and delicious preserve is low calorie and tell us they had to look twice at the label to believe their eyes. *Helen & Eric:* Delicious, fruity taste that makes for a great peanut butter and jelly sandwich.
Availability: Online

PEANUT BUTTER

✱ Peanut Butter
Better'N Peanut Butter
Better'N Peanut Butter
www.betternpeanutbutter.com
Bottom Line: 100 calories per serving (2 tbsp)
Details: One Yummy Hunter, on his doctor's recommendation, cut his fat intake. Thanks to this product, he can still enjoy peanut butter. Another adds that her Weight Watchers lecturer brought it in, and one taste told her peanut butter was back on the menu! *Helen & Eric:* It has a sweeter taste than peanut butter. Delish!
Availability: Supermarkets and health food stores

Peanut Butter
Dixie Diners Club, Beanit Butter
Dixie USA, Inc.
800-233-3668 www.dixiediner.com
Bottom Line: 170 calories per serving (2 tbsp)
Details: Yummy Hunters on the Atkins Diet say this product enables them to eat peanut butter and saves them precious carbs. *Helen & Eric:* Tastes like the real deal to us.
Availability: Online and ordering at www.gethealthyamerica.com

TOMATO

Pomodoro
The Silver Palate, Pomodoro, Sun-Dried Tomato Spread
The Silver Palate
201-568-0110 www.silverpalate.com
Bottom Line: 35 calories per serving (2 tbsp)
Details: Yummy Hunters tells us they love this delicious spread. They put it on crackers for hors d'oeuvres and serve it to company. *Helen:* I spread it on toast with shredded light mozzarella on top. *Eric:* Old world flavor, new world calorie count.
Availability: Supermarkets and online

YOGURT SPREADS

* Strawberry
Brummel & Brown, Creamy Fruit Spread, Simply Strawberry
Unilever Best Foods
800-735-3554 www.brummelandbrown.com
Bottom Line: 50 calories per serving (1 tbsp)
Details: Yummy Hunters rave it's like butter, cream cheese and jelly wrapped into one. *Helen:* I've got my entire family eating it, and everyone says it's simply delicious. *Eric:* Start your spreading, now!
Availability: Supermarkets

* Yogurt
Brummel & Brown, Spread Made with Yogurt
Unilever Best Foods
800-735-3554 www.brummelandbrown.com
Bottom Line: 45 calories per serving (1 tbsp)
Details: *Helen:* Eric's son's mother-in-law Fran turned him onto this. We spread it on toasted English muffins, and it melted and filled all the little crevices. Its flavor is a cross between butter and yogurt, and it's great. *Eric:* I put it on practically everything.
Availability: Supermarkets

To feel "fit as a fiddle" you must tone your middle.

TOPPINGS

Syrups, Whipped Toppings

Eric and I love toppings, but unless you're adding real honest-to-goodness flavor, we'd rather go topless.

SYRUPS

* Caramel
Smucker's, Fat Free, Caramel, Sundae Syrup
J.M. Smucker's Co.
888-550-9555 www.smuckers.com
Bottom Line: 100 calories per serving (2 tbsp)
Details: Yummy Hunters really recommend this product if you're a caramel lover. They say they put it over diet chocolate ice cream and it's delish.
Helen & Eric: Be careful, you can really pour on the calories with this scrumptious syrup.
Availability: Supermarkets and online

* Chocolate
Hershey's, Chocolate, Lite Syrup
Hershey's Foods Corp.
800-468-1714 www.hersheys.com
Bottom Line: 50 calories per serving (2 tbsp)
Details: Yummy Hunters rave this is their favorite chocolate syrup. They love to put it in a blender with eight ounces of fat-free milk and three ice cubes and have themselves a delicious milkshake.
Helen & Eric: The syrup is great. We poured some over angel food cake and heard heaven's choir singing, "Chocolate, oh glorious chocolate!"
Availability: Supermarkets

✳ Chocolate
Walden Farms, Calorie Free, Chocolate Syrup
Walden Farms, Inc.
800-229-1706 www.waldenfarms.com
Bottom Line: 0 calories per serving (2 tbsp)
Details: Yummy Hunters swear it tastes like the real thing. They put it on diet frozen yogurt as well as diet ice cream. They even pour it on some of their low-cal bars. *Helen:* A bit of advice: Use sparingly. In our excitement, we poured too much on the frozen yogurt and there was a bitter aftertaste. Once we got the proportions down, it was heavenly. *Eric:* Help me, for I have sinned!
Availability: Supermarkets, health food stores and online

✳ Ginger
The Ginger People, Stem Ginger in Syrup
Royal Pacific Foods
800-551-5284 www.gingerpeople.com
Bottom Line: 80 calories per serving (1 oz)
Details: Yummy Hunters use it sparingly on ice cream and cakes and it makes for an exotic dessert. *Helen:* You can't get this flavor anywhere else, so we think it's so worth the calories. We put it on diet vanilla ice cream and transformed that snack into an oriental delight. *Eric:* I'm a fool for ginger, and when I first tasted this I went into ginger arrest. The chunks are huge; the syrup, thick and gooey—my God, is it good!
Availability: Online

✳ Hot Fudge
Smucker's, Hot Fudge, Light Toppings
J.M. Smucker's Co.
888-550-9555 www.smuckers.com
Bottom Line: 90 calories per serving (2 tbsp)
Details: One Yummy Hunter confides that at night she and her husband keep their love alive by dunking strawberries into this hot fudge. *Helen & Eric:* We microwaved it and put it on ice cream. Need we say more?
Availability: Supermarkets and online

✳ Maple Butter
Country Cupboard, Maple Butter Flavored Syrup
Country Cupboard
800-382-3267   www.countrycupboard.com
Bottom Line: 10 calories per serving (¼ cup)
Details: *Helen & Eric:* We were thrilled when we discovered this delicious-tasting maple syrup. We had absolutely no idea it contained no fat, no sugar, no cholesterol and no sodium. That's a lot of no's for something we say yes to when it comes to choosing a syrup.
Availability: Online

✳ Pancake Syrups
Walden Farms, Calorie Free, Pancake Syrups
Walden Farms, Inc.
800-229-1706   www.waldenfarms.com
Bottom Line: 0 calories per serving (¼ cup)
Details: When Yummy Hunters who love Walden Farms' products discovered this light pancake syrup, it immediately became their number one choice. *Helen:* Sweet and no bitter aftertaste and just wonderful on waffles. Great on pancakes, too. *Eric:* It may be light on calories, but it's big on flavor. As far as I'm concerned, any way you use it, it stacks up to be one delicious syrup.
Availability: Supermarkets, health food stores and online

✳ Syrup
Log Cabin, Sugar Free, Low Calorie Syrup
Pinnacle Foods Corporation
www.pinnaclefoods.com
Bottom Line: 35 calories per serving (¼ cup)
Details: Yummy Hunters embrace low-cal pancakes and waffles and tell us this is the tops when they're looking for the right syrup. *Helen:* A sweet way to deliciously top off pancake and waffles. *Eric:* I don't miss the sugar and I certainly don't miss the calories. Another childhood favorite that's as good as the original.
Availability: Supermarkets

WHIPPED TOPPINGS

✳ Cool Whip
Kraft, Cool Whip, Lite
Kraft Foods, Inc.
800-538-1998 www.kraftfoods.com
Bottom Line: 20 calories per serving (2 tbsp)
Details: Yummy Hunters say they put Cool Whip on every dessert from fat-free cake or fruit to a diet chocolate muffin. They confess it makes them feel like they're eating a fancy dessert. *Helen:* We have a confession to make, too. We ate it right out of the container! *Eric:* This is one cool whip.
Availability: Supermarkets

Grandma started walking for her health when she was 60. She's now 97 and we don't know where the heck she is!

YOGURT

DELICIOUSLY CREAMY, rich and satisfying, this cultured creation has come a long way, baby.

———————

∗ Apple
Dannon, Light 'n Fit, Fiber With Fiber Apples
Dannon Company, Inc.
800-326-6668 www.dannon.com
Bottom Line: 70 calories per serving (4 oz)
Details: Yummy Hunters say they have trouble getting enough fiber in their diets and can't thank Dannon enough for this delicious treat. *Helen:* The sweetness of apples adds to this unique blending of yogurt and fiber. *Eric:* This tasty yogurt is the apple of my eye.
Availability: Supermarkets

∗ Apricot Mango
Horizon Organic, Fat Free Apricot Mango
Horizon Organic Dairy, Inc.
888-494-3020 www.horizonorganic.com
Bottom Line: 140 calories per serving (6 oz)
Details: Yummy Hunters say it satisfies their sweet-tooth cravings. They love the tropical taste. *Helen:* We loved it. I tasted the apricot, Eric the mango. *Eric:* Go figure?
Availability: Health food stores

* Black Cherry
Stonyfield Farm, Fat Free, Black Cherry
Stonyfield Farm
800-776-2697 www.stonyfield.com
Bottom Line: 130 calories per serving (6 oz)
Details: Yummy Hunters love the smooth texture and authentic black cherry flavor. One mixes this yogurt with a serving of Fiber One cereal and created a new taste sensation, adding excitement to her diet plan. *Helen:* Terrific fruit flavor makes this yogurt a real treat. *Eric:* Perfect size, perfect taste, perfect everything. Thank you, Yummy Hunter, for the Fiber One tip.
Availability: Supermarkets, health food stores, groceries and convenience stores; store locations online

* Blueberry Patch
Yoplait, Light, Blueberry Patch
General Mills
800-967-5248 www.yoplaitusa.com
Bottom Line: 140 calories per serving (6 oz)
Details: Yummy Hunters rave about the plump, juicy blueberries. They tell us they put a serving into the freezer so it takes them longer to eat. *Helen & Eric:* Nice idea. Very cool way to eat this yogurt.
Availability: Supermarkets

* French Vanilla
Stonyfield Farm, French Vanilla Fat Free Yogurt
Stonyfield Farm
800-776-2697 www.stonyfield.com
Bottom Line: 140 calories per serving (6 oz)
Details: Yummy Hunters rave this is their favorite vanilla yogurt and their number one choice when starting a new diet. *Helen:* Great natural vanilla flavor, wonderfully creamy texture. *Eric:* You can eat this yogurt all the time. I do. But then again, I'm French.
Availability: Supermarkets, health food stores, groceries and convenience stores; store locations online

* Key Lime Pie
Yoplait, Whips, Key Lime Pie
General Mills
800-967-5248 www.yoplaitusa.com
Bottom Line: 140 calories per serving (6 oz)
Details: Yummy Hunters declare this is the most refreshing yogurt they've every had. *Helen:* Frothy yogurt mixes well with the outstanding key lime flavor. A great after-dinner palate cleanser. *Eric:* This is another one of the most unique and distinctive products we've come across. Truly delicious!
Availability: Supermarkets

* Peach
Dannon, Light 'n Fit Creamy, Peach
Dannon Company, Inc.
800-326-6668 www.dannon.com
Bottom Line: 100 calories per serving (6 oz)
Details: Yummy Hunters say they always keep this yogurt on hand at the office. It's filled with a great peach flavor and it's only 2 points on Weight Watchers. *Helen:* The fresh taste of peaches gives this creamy yogurt a wonderful burst of flavor. I added fresh strawberries to create a fruit sensation. *Eric:* It's so peachy, it makes our taste buds salivate just thinking of it.
Availability: Supermarkets

* Strawberry
Silk, Cultured Soy, Strawberry
Whitewave, Inc.
www.silkissoy.com
Bottom Line: 160 calories per serving (6 oz)
Details: Yummy Hunters who are lactose intolerant are challenged when it comes to foods to eat, and when dieting, it's twice as hard. They are overjoyed to discover Strawberry by Silk, with its sweet and juicy taste. *Helen & Eric:* The strawberry flavor is mouth watering, and the texture is smooth and creamy.
Availability: Supermarkets and health food stores

* Strawberry Banana
Dannon, Light'n Fit Smoothie, Strawberry Banana
Dannon Company, Inc.
877-326-6668 www.dannon.com
Bottom Line: 80 calories per serving (7 oz)
Details: Yummy Hunters say it's creamy and fruity and, for 80 calories, it fills them up any time of the day. *Helen & Eric:* Thick and Yummy with a true, tropical flavor.
Availability: Supermarkets

* Wild Berry
Stonyfield Farm, Light, Smoothie, Wild Berry
Stonyfield Farm
800-776-2697 www.stonyfield.com
Bottom Line: 130 calories per serving (1 bottle)
Details: Yummy Hunters say it's creamy yogurt with tasty berries. Another add it's delicious in every way. *Helen:* So good, I drank it straight out of the container. *Eric:* You may come in a new light version, but you're still my treasured "old smoothie." Yum, yum.
Availability: Supermarkets, health food stores, groceries and convenience stores; store locations online

I had to quit jogging for health reasons. My thighs were rubbing together so much, my underpants caught on fire.

_____
_____
_____
_____
_____

_____
_____
_____
_____
_____

_____
_____
_____
_____
_____

_____
_____
_____
_____
_____

INDEXES

Company and Product Index

Food Index

Company and Product Index

Fiber with Fiber Apples, 271
Strawberry Banana Smoothie, 26, 274
Dean Foods, Inc.
Bordens, Creamora, Fat Free, Non Dairy
Creamer, 122
Chunky Blue Cheese Salad Dressing, 227
International Delight, Butter Pecan Creamer, 123
Non-Dairy Creamer, 122
Del Monte Foods
Lite Fruit and Gel, Peaches in Strawberry-
Banana Gel, 144
Mandarin Orange Segments in Light Syrup, 142
Peaches, Strawberry, Banana Gel, 147
Deli Select, Thin Sliced, Smoked Turkey Breast, 169, 218
Delicious Fat Free
Blueberry Corn Muffin, 189
Dentyne, Ice, Sugarless Gum, Wintergreen, 154
Devonsheer, Mini Bagel Snacks, Garlic, 116
Diet Snapple
Lemonade Iced Tea, 28
Orange Carrot, 24
Plum-A-Granate Iced Tea, 28
Dijon and Honey with Lemon Juice Marinade, 238
Dill Mustard Grilling Sauce, 238
Dixie USA, Inc.
Beanit Butter, 264
Dole
Pineapple Chunks in Pineapple Juice, 145
Dr. Brown's, Diet Cream Soda, 27
Dr. Praeger's
California Burgers, Veggie Royale, 53
Fish Fillets, 134
Veggie Pizza Burgers, 52, 206
Drake's Coffee Cakes, 56
Dryer's Grand Ice Cream, Inc.
Skinny Cow Bar, Cookies 'N Cream, 16
Vanilla/Chocolate Ice Cream Sandwich, 164
Vanilla/Chocolate, Vanilla/Strawberry Ice
Cream Sundae Cups, 164
Duncan Hines (Kellogg's All-Bran Muffins)
Blueberry, 189

Galaxy Nutritional Foods
Garden Spot Distributor
Gatorade Company, The
General Mills, Inc. (Nature Valley)
George E. Delallo Co., Inc
George Weston Bakeries, Inc.
Gladstone Food Products Co., Inc.

❯T

T. Marzetti Co.
    Cardini's Fat Free, Caesar Dressing, 227
Tabatchnick, Fine Food, Inc.
    Cabbage Soup, 251
    Frenchman's Onion Soup, 257
    Vegetarian Chili, 83
Taco Shells (Old El Paso), 43
Taste of Thai
    Peanut Salad Dressing Mix, 231
    Spicy Thai Peanut Bake, 242-243
Tazo
    Chai, 33
Teeccino Caffe, Inc.
    Chocolate Mint, Caffeine Free, Herbal Coffee, 31
Terra Chips, Sweet Potato, 91
Terra Vegetable Chips, Zesty Tomato, 93
T.G.I. Fridays. See **H.J. Heinz**
Thai Kitchen, Rice Noodle Bowl, Mushroom Medley, 180
Thai Munchees, 7
Thai Peanut Meatless Jerky, 169
Thai, Stir-Fry (Amy's), 187
Thin Additives
    Cranberry Almond Thins, 110
Thin Crisps, Baked Soy Chips, White Cheddar, 92
Thomas'
    English Muffins, 42
      Original, 42
3 Diamonds, Whole Oysters, 135
TLC, Original 7 Grain Crackers, 117
Toasted BBQ Soy Nuts, 195
Tofu
    Miso Soup, 259
    Scramble in a Pocket Sandwich, 187
    Shirataki (House), 246
    Vegetable Lasagna (Amy's), 188
Tofutti Brands, Inc.
    Cream Cheese, Better Than Cream Cheese, 262
Tom-Toms, Turkey Snacks Stick, 170, 221
Tootsie Roll Industries, Inc.
    Tootsie Roll Pops, 64
Topps Company
    Bazooka, Sugarless, Bubble Gum, 151

Food Index

ABOUT THE AUTHORS

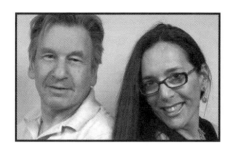

Helen Brand is a NASM certified personal trainer and diet coach with over 20 years of experience. She is also a AAAI/ISMA certified group exercise instructor. She has worked with people of all ages, in groups and one on one. She especially enjoys working with senior citizens and watching them become mentally and physically revitalized and renewed. She practices yoga and kickboxing and works out on a daily basis.

Eric Robespierre is a screenwriter, playwright and documentary film director. He has also been an award-winning advertising copywriter and co-owner of a Web design firm. His humorous take on life is the hallmark of all his creative endeavors. He practices meditation and, because of this book, has established an exercise routine; otherwise, Helen's threat to force him to join her senior citizens' class will be enforced.

Helen can be reached by e-mail at
Helen@romaxpublishing.com

Eric can be reached by e-mail at
Eric@romaxpublishing.com

The authors invite you to visit www.yummyhunters.com for product updates, information on how to become a Yummy Hunter as well as general diet and food information, gift ideas and promotions.

Invoice

ROMAX Romax Publishing LLC
PUBLISHING P.O. Box 2290, Halesite, NY 11743
Phone: 888-296-3913
Fax: 631-424-4644

Date	Invoice No.
08/21/06	1725

Bill To

Martha Ann Thompson
1435 Bowman Rd.
Lawrenceville GA 30045

Ship To

Same